T0088462

THE
Erotic Fire
OF THE
Unattainable

THE
Erotic Fire
OF THE
Unattainable

*Aphorisms on Love, Art, and
the Vicissitudes of Life*

BY GAY WALLEY

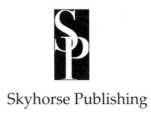

Skyhorse Publishing

First Skyhorse Publishing edition 2015

Skyhorse Publishing books may be purchased in bulk at special discounts for sales promotion, corporate gifts, fund-raising, or educational purposes. Special editions can also be created to specifications. For details, contact the Special Sales Department, Skyhorse Publishing, 307 West 36th Street, 11th Floor, New York, NY 10018 or info@skyhorsepublishing.com.

Skyhorse® and Skyhorse Publishing® are registered trademarks of Skyhorse Publishing, Inc.®, a Delaware corporation.

Visit our website at www.skyhorsepublishing.com.

10 9 8 7 6 5 4 3 2 1

Library of Congress Cataloging-in-Publication Data is available on file.

Cover design by Ashley Lau
Cover photo credit Luciano Fileti

ISBN: 978-1-62914-651-5
Ebook ISBN: 978-1-62914-934-9
Printed in China

"And if the flower
flowers
let it by all means
in itself
flower."

—Theodore Enslin

Acknowledgments

Iwish to thank David B for being with me when I started this in his apartment in Essex, and Terese Svoboda and the late Sondra Spatt Olsen who were my fellow travelers with the pen, who always offered the most valuable insight and encouragement. And to Murphy Lewis Pranlan-Descours and her mother, who first saw something in this and had the courage to bring it forward.

And to Chris Fortunato and Julie Ganz, my esteemed editor, who kept it moving and brought valuable insight to the work, too. Thank you.

Contents

Love	1
Women	15
Love	27
Art	49
Friends and Family	69
Work	77
Rebellion	99
Geography	109
Art	125
Against Society	141
Vicissitudes	161
Spirituality	171
The Future	195

Love

WHY WOMEN FIGHT PIRATES

A woman is captured by a pirate. After all, men do put women on their rafts and bear off to sea with them. The woman must entice and seduce her pirate for fair treatment. He has the power, it is his rickety boat she is living on, and she loves her pirate, yes, she loves his dark loneliness, his individuality, but all the while she is planning her escape onto a God ship, a ship of collective love.

A real woman will not be content with one man. With one man, she will rage, eat into herself and him. She will jump off the pirate ship onto a ship that is gracefully billowing with sails of humanity and the caring of, a ship full of love, of fools. She will not stay isolated in one man's private war with his maleness.

A HANDSOME MAN

I am in love with an unusually handsome man. He is tall and has wide shoulders. A head like a lion. Piercing green-blue eyes. Almost mad. People talk about his looks as a topic. I have become the plain one, the one sitting next to the beacon. I am the smaller stone. I set him off.

I spend the morning thinking about my lover's handsomeness, his blue eyes, his perfect chin and cheekbones, his lips, his tall Greek body. Constantly, I wonder, is there a Faustus underneath this perfect physique? Does he make and talk love so perfectly to hide a lack of feeling? I worry while falling more in love with him.

My lover wears a tan sweater and tan pants. A blue shirt. He was in special forces in Vietnam, a war hero. His blue eyes have flecks of gun chrome in them.

My lover asks me, "Do I look alright?"

He says, "Hi sweetheart" to people he hardly even knows. "Hello dear."

Rivers of watchfulness go up and down my back.

Last night I had dinner with a former suitor who drinks. "We're going to party, right?" he asked as we wait for our table. I tell him I hate that teenage expression. He says he hates it himself, but he passes the bar intimately. At dinner, I tell him my lover is refinding his soul, after Vietnam, prison, women, money. My former suitor says my lover, whom he has never met, never had a soul to begin with. I come home sad and ask my lover, using other words, if he has a soul. He says, "Yes, and it belongs to you."

Faustus would be this quick.

Still in the flush of new love, I wait for my lover's phone call. When I see a fourteen-year-old girl, I know what longing awaits her.

My lover's tallness, khaki pants, white shirt. A plantation owner and I the ensconced slave.

My lover in a black raincoat. He spreads his arm out for me, as if he is an umbrella.

My lover leaves a message at my office: Do you have any idea how much I love you?

My lover is too smooth to be didactic, too clever to antagonize. He prides himself on not being known: not knowing that refusing to be known eventually becomes boring.

My lover says he wants love, tenderness, and sexuality. He says that I provide that. Are these statements from Rod McKewan?

The thrill of being a hero. My lover was one in Vietnam, rode huge waves in Hawaii, made a

❦ *16* ❧

fortune with his illegal businesses. But when we talk it out, it turns out he simply wanted to die.

My lover sent me a love note this morning telling me he is totally in love with me. Do these words of love come easily, as if he is an actor? I ask him sometimes when he declares his love, I say, "What movie did that come from?"

I tell my lover that he is Finnish ice. He says he has never been frightened, which is the lie of the abused. Finnish ice killing in Vietnam, Finnish ice with booze and cocaine and too much money, Finnish ice locked down with no warmth in prison. "You need to be thawed," I say. He agrees, passing his cold blue eyes casually over me.

It is I who am being thawed.

I realize I can articulate what I want and per-haps even receive it with my lover, if only I can be sure he interests me.

I say to my friend, "Well, my lover is like a dog."

"In his blind devotion," my friend concurs.

"No," I say, "I mean in the way he has undifferentiated thoughts."

My lover puts his easel together anxiously and strongly, as if putting together his future.

I cannot keep my hands and kisses off my lover. He says, "Do you think we have chemistry?" I want to eat him up. I take bites out of him. He says soon he will make me sexually voracious, that I will undress him as soon as I see him.

"I redid your ground wire," he says.

I say, "Thank you."

"As if you know what that is," he laughs.

I kiss his chest and stomach. I pull him inside me. I eat with him and I hold his hand in the sunlight. I rub his leg and ankle with my own ankle as we sit side by side. I laugh with him.

My lover says, "Sometimes I think you want to be with no one." Obviously, I am only fooling myself with these charades.

What will we have in common, I ask my lover, when we have exhausted love as a subject?

My lover was married to a famous singer. He drove Porsches that she paid for. He said he worked hard when he was with her. *As hard as a housewife does*, I thought.

It is romantic: a war hero, a prisoner, a man who is athletic, a lover, a dancer. Romantic.

I ask him, "Where is your mind?"

He had many women. He knew what they wanted to hear and feel.

So he is a hero, to men on battlefields and in prison uprisings. To women, he has been a hero of lust and romance, then a thorn.

THE WISDOM OF EX-HUSBANDS

I left my ex-husband because he never made love to me. We were three. My husband, myself, and his anger. Perhaps four. My anger too. A youthful marriage.

I call my ex-husband just for the familiarity of it. He is working on the rigging of his boat and is about to take a sauna. I find these rituals of his moving. My ex has a focus that I admire. That focus is something I can touch down against.

I ask my ex-husband how he handles the loneliness. "I keep busy," he says.

My lover says it is not normal to miss your husband so. I disagree. I failed at knowing how to live in his life, but I never stopped loving who he is.

My ex returns my call last night. He is exhausted but has put a mast on his boat. He is ecstatic. "My mistress," he says. "You better go to sleep," he says, "to get ready for work tomorrow."

I ask my ex whom he went to the movie with. "Alone," he lies. "Good," I say. "You have to be faithful to me all your life."

My tall ex-husband with his long legs. It seems as if he towers over everyone. But it's just the way he looks down at me.

My ex calls and says most surprisingly to me, "You're the best." Only a week ago he told me, "I hated living with you."

The phone man, who was here working, calls me, asking if I found his screwdriver. Everything male reminds me of my ex-husband, not my lover.

My ex-husband said when he was five he loved a certain picture in a book. He began to cut the book up for the picture and then realized he had destroyed the book to get what it was he wanted.

My ex did not like my friends. I do not like many of them myself, but they are the people I have chosen to go through my processes with.

My ex says, "People don't analyze things like you do. Most people just do what the person next to them is doing."

My ex checks his boat continually to see if it is alright. I wish I was his boat.

When I see men walking the street who are the same age as my husband was when he was with me, I long for him. This, I know, will be true, even when my ex-husband is old and looks nothing like the men I look at, searching for him.

My ex is sailing to Cuba with a friend. He calls me from a dock in Block Island to tell me he has migraines, sea sickness on the boat. The Captain is worried, "slightly annoyed" is how my ex puts it. It is my ex, I venture, who is slightly annoyed at showing weakness.

I race down the street, my coat flapping, and send an imaginary kiss to my ex-husband who is on the sea to Cuba. I can see his face as he receives it. The surprise of it.

No word from my ex-husband in Cuba. He is acting like an ex-husband.

A friend says yesterday, "You really love your ex, don't you?" I am reading papers as he asks, and I say, "Yes, I do," and I say nothing more.

My ex has lunch with me when he gets back. We discuss Cuba, how the Captain was punitive and strict with him, how my book has been received. I invite him to spend the weekend, and he refuses. He has to get back to his bills, something he has never been the least interested in.

Did he visit me yesterday as a man does his mother? Many say that is the most erotic of bonds.

As he came up the stairs, he ran into my landlady. "I am visiting my ex-wife," he booms out. What is he trying to tell us all?

"How is my ex?" he asks as he enters the door.

I go to sleep last night aware that my ex is having a party for his birthday and he has not invited me. I can see the intensity in his face as he shucks the oysters, as he drops the lobsters in the boiling water. I can hear his laughter.

Divorced women call me and explain with such aggression how their husbands abandoned them. I feel as if I am being shelled as I listen to their voices. Personally, in my divorce, I went right to the existential grief.

What were those unkind things I did? I was unfaithful mentally, quick to end most arguments with, "Well, maybe we should split up." I was cold during sex because we were so involved out of bed. There had to be somewhere we kept our distance.

My ex hated eating out as much as I forced us to, but he did enjoy looking at the waitresses.

I'd say, "Can I read you this?" "Not right now," he answered.

People I run into on the street do not ask me about him anymore.

I long for his long legs. They held me up.

I long for his mock impatience that began as true impatience and then became a parody of itself.

We were not a couple like others I meet, who have good jobs that they stay at for years, with benefits and salaries that increase. No, we lived on a thread, and the strength of that thread bound us to each other.

As subversives, we kept taking the scissors out.

I do not tell my ex anymore every rejection or victory I experience. I am now alone, which I thought I wanted.

I am a fool.

"When I could have used a wife, I could not support one; when I could support one, I no longer needed any."

—Kant

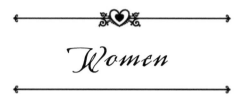

Women

SEX

Women go by in the street wearing skirts that look like slips. Freud said that without sexual desire, nothing happens. No connections, not even business ones, transpire. These women know that.

My friend asks me to describe the best sex I ever had. We are driving late at night, a six-hour drive, and she thinks this discussion will keep us awake. I find the question similar to being asked the best book you have ever read. The best piece of music. I answer her saying that some writers, to carry the analogy, have an unusual use of language. Others have a great narrative. So I go on to describe one man who frequently let himself into my apartment at four in the morning to make love to me. Dream sex was how I explained it to her. She told me about a man with a banana penis. It was amazing, she said. The curve and its effect. I learn by talking to her. I have that rare occasion when I can compare myself to another woman. Only another man can compare you to another woman. I learn that I am passionate, responsive, available but shy, lacking in self-confidence. What strikes me is that this is what I am like out of bed.

I told my friend last night that sex for me is about imagination. That vaginal orgasms are achieved through imagination. "Of what?" a man asks me. The imagination of being desirable, and of desiring.

And yet once I say these words, I am proved wrong. Vaginal orgasms are achieved also by a man knowing how to move. Inside your body, it seems, or inside your mind.

I can't believe men and women are together just for sex. It gets repetitious.

My lover, when making love, focuses on pleasing me, not on his own fire. But the pleasure in sex is in meeting the phallic fire of the man. Pleasure for itself is somewhat uninteresting. We have thousands of autoerotic ways to give ourselves pleasure. The real engagement is with fire.

Sometimes I cannot have an orgasm, or don't want to, so that I can stay tuned to my lover's body.

My lover tells me I am good in bed except that I have claws, I do not know how to work my hands well. My hands are intellectual, used to describe concepts, abstract and quick; inept at making packages, scratching another's back, or giving pleasure. My hands think.

And are often noticed, like a set of eyes, for their articulateness.

My ex-husband would have said I was cold. Many men have said that because the first and primary skill I have developed is distance.

I read in books of people who make love for hours. This I have never done, just like I have never worked on anything for hours. I scurry in out and out of things, intensely there for short periods.

My lover, who has had many lovers, claims to enjoy this best, this having sex with a woman he loves. He finds more pleasure in this than the hungry athleticism of body to body. Especially now that he is middle-aged.

My lover, who . . . himself, is intense and skilled in bed, but repetitive.

My ex-husband never really cared to help me become responsive to him. He wanted me to be vulnerable to him while he maintained a kind of distance of his own. But the Greeks knew that eros is "absence." Distance, the ultimate aphrodisiac.

My husband was, however, creative in bed, because I forced him to objectify me.

My lover, the sexual athlete, uses only one position, the missionary, because, I think, he needs that intimacy and reassurance. The eroticism for him is my presence.

WOMEN AND BEAUTY

Old women sit outside having coffee and staring off. They are completely desexed. In their men's pants and short cropped grey hair, they overstate their leaving of the sexual theatre. And yet I have friends of sixty, perhaps even the same age as these women I watch, who've dyed their hair blonde, who dress as women still, ergo to attract, and enjoy their own beauty. Which is real? I suppose these women having their coffees were never the divas to begin with.

A friend tells me yesterday, "Well, you are not beautiful. Your lover will love you for your depth and charm." I feel a knife go through me. But why should I need to be told I am beautiful? Because, left to myself, I sink into seeing myself as a beast.

I run into another friend, and she tells me this obsession with feeling ugly is a transference. I am seeing myself through the eyes of my mother, who left me. Also, with my divorce, there is no one to replace my mother's unaffected eyes. I am the Beast.

This morning upon further reflection I realize that the Beast in *Beauty and the Beast* became beautiful once he expressed his anger. The anger curled inside is what makes you feel hideous.

Some of us even look at the aged as if they failed. How dare they not be beautiful? How dare they remind us of our own powerlessness against staying beautiful ergo lovable?

My lover tells me most people feel unlovable. "Why?" I ask, just to hear his thoughts. "Failures of love," he says. He does not yet speak in the personal.

It is not beauty that makes me love a man. It is his openness (ergo his desire), his vulnerability (how he hurts), his imagination (how he will take). His ability to love and be loved. This is beauty.

My lover says we like to blame failures of love on our exterior. Which is ridiculous. But once when my first husband was not speaking to me and living separately from me, before we were married, I longed, oh I longed to have longer hair for him. Perhaps I thought growing my hair for him would be a manageable surrender to the relationship.

I tell my lover that I am bringing my best friend with me to visit him next weekend. A clever, witty, generous woman who is short and stocky and not beautiful. Perhaps ugly, I cannot tell. To me, she is beautiful. Her sensuality, her friendship, her wit all shine through. I say, "Let's fix her up with your friend." "No," he says. "She is not so and so's type." I am desperately wounded by this. She is a better woman than the beauties my lover's friends waste their time with. I am wounded, as if it was me he rejected.

I have known many women who are not beautiful who believe they are. Their mothers must have doted on them. I have known many beautiful women who pay little attention to themselves. Their mothers must have doted on them.

Women feel a pang of sadness for a young girl as she follows her parent down the street. What she will go through.

One's own beauty is an homage to life, a participation in it. It is essential to find one's own beauty, to offer it to the gods in thanks. To honor God's ecology. To go against one's own beauty is to indulge in narcissistic anger at not getting what one wants. It is not honoring what has been put before us.

Why we love beauty: We know it is a thankfulness.

A man I know is fixing my VCR and does not give up. I would be inclined to throw all this old technology out and buy new machinery with money I do not have. He patiently works, adjusting this, fiddling with that, insisting it will work. This is a gift I do not know why I deserve. Perhaps he sees beauty in me.

A man ill-suited to me seems attracted to me and I to him. "But we have nothing in common," I say to a friend. "Yes, but he is masculine and you are feminine," she replies.

A beautiful young woman sits at the bar. It is I who stare at her, not the men. The men surprise me by looking at me, someone middle-aged whom they think might be desperate enough to accept them despite their desperation.

This same friend who three years after her divorce is still grieving worries about being ten pounds overweight. She misses cooking for a man and thus cooks for herself. We agree that much of overeating, for a woman, is anger. I say, "You know that all women think they are ten pounds overweight." She says there is so much shame around all this for her that she has avoided her young lover purely because of her ten pounds. I say, "When you lie down they can't tell the difference." But it is about something else, this guilt at not being sylph-like. Are we ashamed that we are not innocent and taut? That we will not be malleable and fully able to believe every lie of unconsciousness? We cannot fool ourselves or them.

I see a young woman with a plump body and she is beautiful. I see a slight flaw in myself and I want to be flogged.

I walk outside for tea on a warm November afternoon and am reminded that life is much fuller than what one's experiences have revealed. Life is beauty, continual beauty unfolding.

"You look beautiful," someone says. "You must be happy." I am too tired to be happy. I look beautiful perhaps because right now I have no time for myself. Perhaps he sees me as beautiful because I am self-forgetful.

"Why do people look at me?" I ask my ex-husband.

"Partially how you look and partially because you need them to," he answers.

"Who acts without desire
Is beauty's ruin and the plague of nations."
—Guy Davenport

Love

THE DISAPPOINTMENTS OF INFIDELITY

I told my friend an affair is a sign of having given up. You believe you cannot get the love you want.

I was in love with my handsome lover when I was with my husband. We never slept together, but we talked on the phone, we wrote letters. It was he I walked with (in my mind) as I did my errands. It was his initials I penned sometimes as doodles. It was a future with him I planned. When I made love with my husband sometimes passionately, I had just seen my platonic lover.

Sometimes I will tell you my husband left me.

Now, I long for my husband, as a lover. I see that the person is irrelevant. One just longs for the Other.

Infidelity is exciting in the moment. A new face saying new words of admiration in a new voice makes it seem as if these words were never said before.

But there is no replacing the texture of a person you live with. They start to transmute into your blood and they cannot be removed.

Some people do stop loving their previous spouse. But I believe that these people never allowed their spouse into their bloodstream to begin with.

But the longing, the longing for the Other is a continual call. One pays no attention to how the Other will fail you.

Sex with a stranger can be exciting, but always cold. You never stop being strangers.

My lover, when he was in prison, said he did not long for sex, for you can have sex with yourself, but he longed for tenderness.

To be known, which the infidel can never be.

There is no doubt that sex with a lover is initially more erotic because it is not held down by the gauze of the marital.

It eventually loses its pleasure because it is not held together by that same gauze.

In infidelity, one asks to still be found beautiful, still alluring, still magical. Ergo not mortal.

Taking a lover as an act of anger at one's spouse is not infidelity, but a misplaced act with the spouse.

Fidelity, however, seems a closing of a door. A closing of a door into a room that may be lovely, but there are some people who cannot close a door.

Some men feel it is their right as men to bed as many women as possible. But these same men come into their fifties wanting to want to be faithful.

Fidelity, their own ability for it, becomes the Other they long for.

So, in their fifties, often they will leave their spouses for the Other, in hopes that with the new woman they can be physically and spiritually faithful.

And usually they achieve this. For, in their fifties, they have learned the sensuality of talking. They think that finally they may have something to say. Their first wives have forgotten how to speak or listen, having so long been ignored.

However, even being listened to and loved by another woman or man will not assuage the pain of the death of a marriage.

The death of a marriage through infidelity feels like a murder. It haunts.

Single men are not usually unfaithful to their girlfriends. They spent too much time winning them. The keeping of the girlfriend becomes the love affair.

THE WAR OF THE SEXES

My friend tells me her husband's lack of intensity is both annoying and relaxing for her. I pray for such generosity.

I like that my lover is vocal about his love. Tells me he will stay with me forever. Always be faithful. That he is sure. It is another way he makes love. I don't have to listen to my own narrative. I have the opportunity with this aggressive man in love to listen to his. In fact, my lover's narrative is kinder to me than my own would be. Perhaps it is for this that I love him.

I spend the weekend with an engaged couple. They are consumed with planning the wedding, the rituals. I take vicarious pleasure in it. My lover asks, "What music would you want at our wedding?" "The theme to Perry Mason," I say, "because you like to cross-examine me so much." "What vows?" he asks. "You could interrogate me." He laughs. We all want so much to be seen.

A man says, "I find you fascinating." We are both embarrassed. Neither of us knows why he would.

In jail, my lover used to joke that the prisoners committed their crimes for women. Yes, for women, and to buck their fathers.

A friend calls and tells me that her husband says they have to work on their relationship.

"What do you mean?" she asks him. "You have to have more sex with me," he says.

A friend sees a movie about French women. "They look like we should look," she says. "As you can hear, the TV is on," she says. Code that her husband is there.

"What about a normal man?" a friend asks me. I wave my hand away, as if there could be one.

Men so willing to listen to, be directed by women.

A man calls and says, "Call me if you need anything. Anything," he affirms.

Creative people seem to go toward, away, toward, away, toward in their marriages. Frieda Kahlo, Diego. Dawn Powell and her husband.

My friend says when she asks her boyfriend how he is, he tells her what is going on in Chechnya. High-class complaining, she calls it.

Almost no personal calls today. That is because it is the day before a holiday, and women, my friends, are busy preparing.

My lover loves to solve problems. Says it is why he likes me.

My lover and I lie down to watch a film, but I want to make love. I kiss him, try to distract him. Finally he switches off the film.

Men do not mind when women are impractical. I am amazed at this.

Men love working with tools. I do not know why.

Women use men as tools.

SUSPICION IN LOVE

I always thought my ex did not love me. He would reply, "I'm here, aren't I?"

I began to look for proof of his lack of love. And then I began to prepare for it. And so I began to leave him.

I send men out to grow up. I insist on it. To these male children, I say, "You go out and conquer Goliath. That's your job."

Being men, they are confused and think they should do as I say. But finally they throw their cross-bow down and say they'd rather play, too.

Our suspicions of course tell so much more about ourselves. When I was married, my husband and my step-sister went out late one country evening to get cigarettes. I imagined them pulling over to the side of the road, overcome with desire, and making love lustfully in the car. And it was true they did not seem to come home right away. When my husband returned to our bedroom, I quietly asked, "How was the drive?" "We had a huge fight," he said, "about my refusing to wear the seat belt."

I am suspicious of stories.

I am suspicious that there is no safety against anything. In the end, Goliath may win. David wins at first, but only for a second, and a great story is born. We all love a hero. But what about when Goliath gets back up?

Battles are won by endurance, resilience, strength of heart, not in momentary epiphanies or brave acts. They are won through stubbornness.

All endings are false. Only death is a true ending. For the dead. And even this morning I lie in bed proving to myself that there are souls. *Even dogs have them*, I tell myself. We are all so different. Thus there might not even be an ending in death.

All endings are false. I divorce and love my husband still. I say I will trust my lover and feel as distrustful of him as I did of men when I was growing up. All is a river moving. Our perception is the water.

I am suspicious that I will disaffect in love. That I will lose interest. That I will not bond. I forget that one is always bonding, even when not liking a person, just by proximity.

Women are taught to conciliate. I am suspicious that I will be caught in someone else's silly life. Not my own silly life, which is bad enough.

LONGING FOR MY EX

I spent eighteen years leaving him. All because I knew I couldn't leave him.

I longed for the edgy feeling I had of always wanting his love. He said he did love me in those days, but like heroin, I always wanted to up the dosage.

I longed for his tall, rangy body that looked beautiful to me constantly.

As I visit my aging mother, the photos of me around her house are with my ex. Those I sent long ago. It used to bother me that those photos were still up, but now I see them as what is emotionally alive in me anyway.

She is now too dotty to put up the photo of me with my lover, which I sent for her amusement. My lover looks like one of her lovers. Perhaps she thought he was.

My ex was always busy with material life, wood, houses, cars, the ocean, nature. As I was busy in my mind.

Saunas, sailing, maps, voyages. I was fired by being near such passion.

I did not know one cannot get over a man like that.

My ex is my first loss that is my fault. My mother's abandonment of me and my father's death were not my fault.

My lover leaves me a message while I am in Europe of how much he loves me. My ex would never do that. He might have called, in the old days, and said, "Who loves you?" Even then, he wanted me to guess.

My lover gives me a banquet of words. Yet, here I am longing for my ex who gave me a banquet of cold constancy.

HOW MY EX NEVER FORGAVE ME FOR MY BAD BEHAVIOR

This morning I drive to work and feel so sad that I never appreciated the tasteful jewelry he gave me. That he had that sense of what suited me exactly.

He tells me not to worry about anything.

Even divorced, he gives me a birthday card saying: To she who is forever young and in my heart.

I try to understand how I did not nurture our love. I come up with confusion.

Now, I urge all my friends to stay married. They complain of boredom, resentments, coldnesses. I say, "Work it through. You have woven something deep. How can you think it can be ripped out?"

At this point, neither of us knows who left whom. There was so much resentment everywhere. We both kept failing each other.

Now I only think how wrong it is not to yield, not to submit, as long as you can still do what is important to you.

And so I tell myself, yield with your lover. Don't make the same mistake. But I see the same old resistances in me. I do not want to move in with my lover. I think about others.

I sent my ex a fable I had written. He never read it.

I no longer know what his passions are. I no longer know what he thinks about. He is speaking words that are unfamiliar to me. He wears clothes I do not know. He laughs at things I do not say.

He is a man who marries. He will love her and be constant.

My intensity irritated my ex. His own was all-consuming. He wanted a woman who would cater to his overwhelming need, and I was too busy catering to mine.

I chastise myself that I was weak with him. I would not let myself know how vulnerable I felt, how much I loved him. I kept a distance. I was counterphobic to our love. Continually I pushed him away, while wanting him to stay.

Finally he took my advice.

ON MARRIAGE

I now know that once you are bonded, once you are committed, you just stay. What Bill Cosby called the secret to a happy marriage: you just go home every night.

Like an occupied country, I was always seceding.

A man with whom I could listen to music.

One fuses with a soulmate but does not necessarily get on better.

My friend last week said she was thinking of leaving her husband. This week they have been so in love, she says, and making love all the time. This is marriage.

There is no greater pleasure than music, than having your nails done, than running into friends on the street. No greater pleasure than learning something new. Marriage must include all this.

I am elated at my freedom. I want to feel the same about my marriage.

To work in one's office, to work, is one's marriage. Why so many men are happy at work. Women of my generation don't admit to it.

I suddenly know I will marry again. When I sit with a new man, I lean toward him. I look at small towns by the sea and imagine me there with him and all his mysteries. I smile as my imaginary second husband walks toward me across the sand.

I can be silent with him. I am almost ready.

I no longer want my ex. He is better off with his new woman. Let her have those difficulties of which I know. They were not ALL my fault.

In other words, and if nothing else I tell you is valuable, this is: the mourning ends.

TALK IN LOVE

I say to my lover, "Well, you're uncommonly handsome. Your dog is. Your daughter is. Wouldn't you like to be with a beautiful woman who matches your family?"

"Listen," he says, "when we were lying down on the floor, and I looked at you—I thought, to me, you are so beautiful." But you couldn't even see me, I think.

He said, "If you leave me I will go back to jail."

"To Jane?" I respond, pretending I misheard him.

"Don't ever leave me," he says.

"But I don't know if we have enough in common." I always say that.

I tell him I will stay with him forever, but I don't believe it. Although I might.

I tell him that I will marry him even while planning to leave him. Because I want to marry him and I don't even know why.

I tell my ex "Who loves you?" "You do," he replies.

My lover tells me that I have been elusive with him. "What are you going to do?" I ask. He says, "Put on more pressure."

I have dinner with my ex, and we talk about politics, people, trips. I have dinner with my lover, and we talk about how I did not pay enough attention to him at a party we went to.

"When will you be back?" I ask as he goes to get food.

"In a few days."

I tell him a friend said that he considers his wife the love of his life. "That's ridiculous," my lover says, "There is no such thing."

"We should do things," he says. "Want to play golf? Canoe?" I shake my head.

"We have to get cigarettes," I say, after we have eaten breakfast. "I know that," he replies.

"Say something romantic," I say.

"Well, we will have just come back from the beach," he says, "when we are seventy, and we'll make love and we'll hold each other like this and I'll tell you that I was wrong. You are the love of my life."

"Pretty good," I say.

"I'll always give you money when you need it," he says. Forgetting that I have always needed it.

"I yell at friends now," my ex says. "Now that I don't have you to yell at."

"You say:
'I fear a man obsessed.'
And I fear one
who is not."

—Theodore Enslin

Art

WRITERS

Why do I wear perfume and lipstick as I write? Indeed the perfume is dripping down my neck. Clearly writing is an erotic act for me.

Dostoyevsky, Balzac, and many nineteenth century novelists wrote about money. How the lack of it or the abundance of it created a person's circumstances, revealed character. Nothing revealed the baldness of character more than the grasping for money. Twenty-first century novelists are slyer and act like it is a dirty secret. It must be because they are keeping its cruel thrall to themselves. No one wants to talk about how we have all been bought.

All books are about our longings and then the brutal discovery of what it is we really long for.

My published book reveals to the world that I became brutal. Anyone can pick it up and know just how brutal.

The advantage to being this psychologically naked is that I can feel the cold and the heat intensely.

What I know deep down is that most people are happy when you receive an unfavorable review.

Hubris. God does not allow it.

My mind switching and switching. That is all it does. From writing to work to love to grief to writing to work.

Why they think artists are charlatans: Matisse cried when someone liked his work, so expectant was he of the opposite. Whitman wrote favorable reviews of his work under assumed names.

Would that I had that energy.

A poet friend says that artists have a character failing of not being generous one to the other. There is some truth to this. It is so difficult because each of us has taken such lashings. The odd one who is generous is an incredible rarity, a jewel.

Nin was and is vilified, even by me. She exposed herself in all her weaknesses. But who am I to dismiss her work like a bad pudding? I would be kinder to a person who made a bad pudding. To a writer, we are quick to draw our swords. As if they are there for our rage and dismissal. Pass me a rotten egg to throw.

I could not listen when a man was speaking this morning. I wanted style in his words, and

only then would I be able to hear the content.
This is how artists live differently.

"You have wonderful descriptions," someone
says. "It's an unusual book." I take that to mean
she didn't like it.

A man calls and says he got my book. He
read the prologue and wants to give me a book
review.

My Ukrainian landlord comes up to fix the
cold water faucet. I enjoy watching his machinations. They are the same we use in writing.
He is either filing an old piece down or using
a wire to reshape or tie together. I pour him a
schnapps.

I fax my monthly bill to my business client.
There is literature and there is the power of this
piece of paper.

A friend calls. He read my book in typescript,
and now he is reading it in print. He does not

believe he read it before. Only now he takes it seriously.

I listen to Leonard Cohen. I play Chopin and Beethoven (badly) on the piano. It is the first time in what seems like months that I have been alone enough to play the keys. I am vaguely remembering what to create means. It is to take energy and make something of it.

I reject Rimbaud's philosophical swings as the extremism of a young romantic, but somehow accept philosophical swings from Nietzche, who tried for rationalism in his changes of heart. Thus, I castigate my own romanticism.

I despise how a writing class can become to some the whole forum. The artist should be foremost an explorer, not a housecat.

The man at breakfast says it is someone else who is writing when he writes, not himself. I have heard this before and I distrust it. To me, that is wanting to kill the ego because you are not able to kill the ego.

I hate when people tell me someone else is writing in my style. As if someone beat me to the punch in being me.

We must face the fact that incredible sadness segues into a need for imagination.

MUSIC

Listening to a virtuoso flute is one way of encountering purity.

Live music blows the dirt out of the psyche and renews it.

The sax player friend I went to hear went home with a young woman at the bar. She is a psychologist who writes poetry. In her taking on all his needs and problems, I feel she is being sacrificed to music.

I am learning the piano. I play a little bit every day, in a most unschooled fashion. I do it as a Zen meditation, a new language. I lose myself in the difficulty of reading music, the new sounds. I understand the pleasure of linguists.

My piano teacher tells me reading music is much harder than reading words. It synchronizes body and mind. It is as difficult as loving.

French classical music—delicate, sensual, a beautiful seduction. Italian music—heavier, more deeply sensual, moving, as in the manner of the Italians where they do not smile unless they are seducing you.

I play the piano while calling Amtrak. The sublime and the prosaic.

Occasionally at dinner in a restaurant, sitting outside, one hears someone practicing his horn. This is good and is what happens. I have yet to hear a flute player. Where are they practicing? In Sufi poetry.

Chopin again. Playing his music makes me want to know him. The teacher said that no one knew the piano like he did, except for perhaps Rachmaninoff.

I practice a Chopin mazurka. It gives me sublime pleasure to fumble through. I treat my life in the same way, searching for the beauty, fumbling through.

To lie down and be quiet. I don't have time so instead I play Barber's String Adagio. Its sadness allows my soul to rest.

Such pleasure to listen to Clifford Jordan and not to talk.

It's odd how the actual playing of music can feel so wooden, so unmusical. Hammering at the ramparts of this spiritual art.

When visitors stay with me and I find myself losing my inner self, I put music on to aright the alchemy of the inner life taking precedent.

If I want to set my spirit free, I put on music very loudly for ten minutes. My spirit flies off with it.

My ex liked music where he could oom pa pa to the beat. He liked the repetitious.

My lover hears music in restaurants and begins shaking his head to it like he is a rag doll.

Sometimes he pulls me to him as if to dance when he hears music. And I do not know if it is the music inspiring him or if he is using the music as an opportunity to pull me toward him.

Men have used music to conquer for centuries. To conquer women and to inspire their own souls to battle.

My ex and I went out to hear music together. If it was classical, I was happy and he was bored. If it was blues, he was happy and I was bored. Music became a weapon of control between us.

My lover says he could not stay with a woman whose speaking voice was not musical.

Laughter can be musical, if you're in the mood. Some people use laughter, however, to intrude, to dominate.

Women and men both listen to female voices when they want to rage inside.

A British newspaper editor used Beethoven to quell his pain when in the hospital. He had a phonograph installed in his room.

A doctor told a friend of mine to listen to Beethoven every day as preventative maintenance for her health.

Music is the wealth of the poor, everywhere. The soul needs it, like it needs God.

People make the mistake of thinking, when they play their music too loud, that they are thus setting free the neighborhood.

LITERATURE

I was out with a writer last night and he talks about the promise of money from his lecture agent, not the mysterious calling of his new book.

A man passing me in the parking lot yells out, "I read your book." I say, "Oh, thank you. How did you like it?" He doesn't answer. Till later he remembers the question and further out in the parking lot, he yells, "I liked it." But what else could he say? I should refrain from the question.

Nonfiction tells me about life, and I appreciate it. Fiction makes me relive my own life more deeply.

Without comment, a friend returns books I lent her to read. Her lack of enthusiasm makes me feel so sad for the authors.

Characters live on in our minds, as old friends. A friend compares me to Holly Go Lightly, as if we know her. I lie in bed and wonder if my marrying my lover is the same as a character in a Somerset Maugham story. I look to this story to guide me, not to what people say to me in real life.

I try to tell myself redemption is an interesting theme for a story. But it isn't. One always suspects a redemption as a bit easy. Not only in literature.

American literature of the twenties and thirties dealt much with the hardship of living. The forties were how to participate in a mad world. The fifties' and sixties' literature became interested in the vagaries and lonelinesses of the mind. The seventies showed how family could stultify. The eighties became preoccupied with dealing with cancer and AIDS. The nineties became madly interested in peoples of different ethnicities. This next century begins a literature sustaining humanity as the antiseptic of technology takes over.

Even in this day of "voices," good literature renders the author's personality silent.
The voice of the work must sing of another.
If the voice sings of itself, it must be intensely
wrestling with the other.

The madness of a character is our own. The
desire for love in a character is our own.

Film actors have become famous authors.
Politicians, too. As if writing a book stamps these
professional chameleons with authenticity.

Books approach the sublime and yet they are
written while workmen wash the windows,
mothers lie in hospitals, and bills plague the
author.

The common truth you can count on a book
to tell you is that there is pain and loss.

Dreams sometimes unfold like complete
books. So much so, one thinks one could write
one's dream as a book. But if one does, the story
does not seem credible. Dreams are the true

stab of the emotional knife (the feeling itself), not the actual way (narrative) the knife goes in.

A writer looks at another writer's work in process to see if he or she has perhaps "opened the vein" of transcendence. We do this, forgetting it is impossible for all of us. None of us are God, although we set out thinking we are.

And yet can we imagine a life without Tolstoy's Natasha? Anna Karenina? Can we imagine a life without Susan Sontag's depiction of AIDS and how it runs through a community of friends? Can we imagine a life without Carver's mishaps? No. They, like our family and countries, run through our veins.

Kafka published only two of his great works in his lifetime. However, he kept working, and now all his works are part of the literary canon. As if he knew.

Fitzgerald and the beautiful losers. He had to get them out of himself.

What are books about? People wanting to break out of themselves. Psychology proposes we can talk ourselves into freedom. Books show how we cannot.

TALENT, WHAT IS IT?

Hundreds of people I know write cleverly, quickly, energetically. But refuse insight. Their withholding is a form of anger.

Many people can sing, play a musical instrument. What is rare is the willingness or the ability to put themselves into it.

Talent seems to me continual engagement between one's craft and the insides of one's nerves.

My boss says, "I attacked the piece you wrote." "With the Marines?" I ask. He does not even hear me, so focused is he on his subject.

I see talent in my friends' writings. There is the artful phrase, always, throughout each paragraph. So what is missing? I admit some of my critical posturing is perhaps a defense against envy, but when you read a great work, all the world, even the envious, are lifted into celebration. What makes work large and necessary is when the craft is maneuvered by the heart.

Most talented people know they have work to get out but do not know they are talented. All they know is they are surprised other people do not bear this same pressure.

Talent demands a life of rebellion against the collective. One keeps oneself separate enough to see. Talent requires a commitment to that.

Talent knows what it has to do. Beethoven knew he had to get his work out, no matter what. He never questioned it. No matter the economic or health difficulties he had, he knew he had to get the music down. Only after he did, could he die.

Talent is not fueled by the desire for money. Money comes to some but not to all the talented.

Talent only insists on the recognition that it contribute to the ocean of talent before and after.

Talent is lonely. Talented people are often rejected, even when they receive adulation. Admiration of talent comes with jealousy and resentment. The talented person is often too naive to understand this.

Talented people secretly believe that being good will reap rewards. That is because talented people believe life has been good to them, even if life has been difficult. Life has made them rich with their need to create.

Talented people may be counterphobic to their own compassion and love, but they know, in their heart, that all work is about love.

They are easy marks for cons and needy people.

Talented people demand intense relationships. They must talk deeply and be emotionally honest at all times. There are no reprieves, no breaks with the talented. If they are not working at their art, they are working in their mind.

Silliness for itself is a waste of time. Many talented people are clowns but only to elicit, from the moment, the freedom of new material. Talented people exhaust the people around them because they want so much connection.

When talented people are left alone, because others cannot sustain such intensity, they turn back to their work, as they always knew they would have to, sad and lonely.

My ex told me I would have been more successful if I had become dependent on him and lived a quieter, smaller life. Had sailed with him and taken more time for my work. But I was not sure that even the pages could have contained my frustration.

The talented person rarely says, "I have to go back to work." Instead she or he says, "We have to break up." The possibilities in solitude are so vast and necessary that they often destroy whatever kindness others may offer.

Some artists, most artists, need the stabilizing lover/spouse so they are free, when working, to walk the dangerous ramparts. It is easier to travel in uncertainty, knowing there is a warm bed waiting that night. Those are the lucky ones who live longer and produce more.

My lover's talent has gone into wooing me. He enjoys speaking words of love, almost as performance art. Even if he is tired or busy, he says, "No, let me go on talking." He wants to create us.

It is hard to part forever from talented people because they live the relationship forever in their mind. Even when it ends, it does not end for them because it has been absorbed as a living entity and acts as a creative fulcrum.

"Do not crush my hand.
Strength will not grasp it.
Deceit will not reach it.
Giving me the
'glad hand.'"

—Theodore Enslin

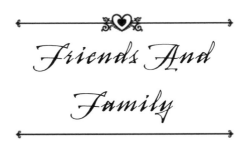

Friends And Family

BEWARE OF GIFTS

My parents had sociopathic tendencies, as do we all. I lavished gifts upon them and the universe to ward off their evil spirits. I behave the same way with my friends. If I lavish you, you will not hurt me. If I stop giving gifts, I will see what evil lies behind the lavishment.

I often give gifts I cannot afford to people who are not even close to me because I cannot give a gift that I myself would not want. It would feel as if I am aggressively insulting them.

When a man gives me a gift, I am always embarrassed. It is never quite what I want. Yet he is kind to give of himself in this way. So there is the vulnerability of pleasure coupled with a slight disappointment. In other words, relationship.

Gifts, like everything else, tell everything about the person giving it. Sometimes one does not want to know that much about the giver, and so the gift hurts in some way. It is another form of fantasy being stripped away.

That's why many men have trouble giving gifts to women. They don't want to be so easily revealed.

Often people who crave kindness, like me, give expensive gifts. People who can never be loved enough give very few and miserly gifts.

FAMILIES

Families, weighed down by their disappointments in one another and the disappointments in themselves as shown to them by family members, walk slowly in groups.

Young men walk quickly, stride out, hungry.

My friend speaks frequently of what she will do when her husband dies. She is unconscious of her repetition. This playing with the image of her widowhood is her way of capturing free-dom in her marriage. She uses these images like others use affairs, platonic or sexual.

I tell my friend last night that I would like to marry again, I who got married at forty-one the first time and had to practically be blackmailed into it. I tell her it is not good to be alone, it is good to share one's troubles, cuddle up on a winter's eve. I tell her this even though I love my alone-ness far more passionately than she loves her married state. What are we really saying? That the idealization of union surpasses any reality.

My Ukrainian landlords come up to look at my swollen door. I cannot close it anymore. The mother and father who own the building come to look. The daughter follows. We talk about buildings. I have never felt more at home than I do here. The building is all family. Not my own, but just the architecture of their family heals me.

I stop in and see my Ukrainian landlords. The seventy-eight-year-old mother is sewing and fixing things for her forty-year-old daughter. That is how they both stay young.

I have no children and have many dinners with young women for whom I am the "wild" mother. And what is it they want from me? That I do not lie to them.

I show my visiting brother a picture of us as children. He looks at himself and says, "What an ugly child." He means, "What a pain-filled child."

Yet he is able to give to his own children. This, rather than killing in war, should be awarded for valor.

I talk nonsense for hours with my niece, a seven-year-old girl. I do it very seriously.

In marriage, the husband is always wrong when trying to do something new.

My brother and his family finally mobilize to see the city. They align their sensitivities, as if four people can. His youngest is happy to be in on any adventure. She can talk to her beanies.

Last night my Ukrainian landlords returned from the country. I helped them carry apples from their trees and bottled water up the stairs. This is the healing part of my day.

My mother's boyfriend in London calls to report on her hip surgery. He answers my questions, "That's right," "No,"—a series of monosyllables. I shoot my questions out rapid fire, as if the speed will obfuscate my helplessness.

My lover has a daughter, but we three do not interact as a family. He does not include her in our activities. "She is busy," he says. I suppose all three of us are so needy for the other, that we cannot share.

Some parents hold hands with their children in the city fearing someone will snatch them away. Another case of "in the eye of the beholder."

A man tells me that during his entire thirty-one-year marriage, he thought he would leave. So few of us are willing to accept ordinary unhappiness.

"Understand—through the stillness,
Act—out of the stillness,
Conquer—in the stillness.
'In order for the eye to perceive color, it must divest itself of all colors.' "

—Dag Hammerskjold

Work

WORK AND ITS PUNISHMENTS

There are some days I take off from work without knowing it. Some days that my mind aborts commerce. I am at my desk but no commerce transpires. A type of internal music has filled me up, and I have to traverse there. To be right-brained is to sustain the demands of dreams, music, fantasy.

One of the young Persian engineers I work with is elegant and witty and kind. I say at a meeting that if I were thirty years younger, I would go for you. He says if he was older, he would go for me. As the meeting progresses, I worry that I have sexually harassed him.

The days are interminable at an office. Stiff clothes. Air conditioning. The hum of computers, printers. Beige walls. The sense of being watched all the time. Office paranoias and conspiracies become the color, the ragged, the human.

The men tease me about eating. I eat ravenously at an office because I would rather be home. I have always longed for a man who could afford to keep me home. When I have met that type, I act my most confused and hostile. Let me sabotage what I will not accept anyway.

A small woman at the office, in prim grey and navy blue dresses, with the bluntest of short blonde hair, admits to having had all kinds of lovers. I call her Liz Taylor and she laughs.

Almost impossible to be creative at an office with the phone ringing, people interrupting, busy work insisting. Equally impossible not to try.

I now remember what was deadening in an office I went to this morning: The walls had no art. Hence the lack of energy.

I am too old really to start a new career but not too old to be open-minded.

To work is to be given the privilege of participating in life. The myriad ideas. The strivings. Humanity.

Being mired in the mundane of business fights the compensating rush to delusional thinking.

Odd to see these men I discuss business with all the time go out to sleazy Western bars and lick a waitress' neck and smile up at her in bliss as she pours the tequila.

Men adore women. The power of it almost shocks me. I androgynize to do business, as I should.

Much of men's posturing for women is performing in front of the other men. Their competitiveness. "I can make the sale and I can get the girl." Men understand this and applaud it.

The company president tells me that he had two important things to do when he got in. I imagine he had to sell off companies, sign complicated contracts. As our conversation continues, he reveals one was an address change. This heartened me.

Male voices defining numbers and sizes, one to the other.

A woman chimes in, No that one is the best.

At the party, the president stops by my table and says, "What are you drinking?" I say, "Nothing, thanks." We make stabs of contact in our attraction.

The president kisses me goodbye at the office party. He is on his way to Asia. I pass him outside in the parking lot, and we silently smile one to the other, shy and reserved.

People come into my office where I am intent at my computer. "Are you working?" they ask.

I am so tired that at dinner I ask an engineer the same question, "Are you excited about getting married?" "You asked me that six times," he said annoyed.

The big boss strolls through the office like a cheetah. I see him from the corner of my eye.

I say, "How are you?" to the secretary. She gives me a long-winded answer from luncheons to workload to irritable bowel syndrome. My mind races away from the conversation like a rat.

The phone rings less in the afternoons. People have completed their to-do lists. The cats sit in the windows.

To have free time is sunlight. Quentin Crisp said that his secret of longevity was not working.

If there is free time, as there is now, the world becomes beautiful. One is able to see the way the sun is falling over the street, feel the warmth. No wonder people who are too busy shop and drink in anguish.

"Why are you here?" the secretary says. "I have to see the president," I say, "for ten minutes. But it's an important ten minutes."

I see a man sitting on a bench in the sun, drinking in the middle of the day. I know he would be happier if he was employed, experiencing all those frustrations. If he was wanted.

The men at work are used to requests from a woman. They wait patiently as I go down my list with them. For a minute, they are at home.

MY BOSS

He never says anything complimentary to me. However, he smiles when we speak. Thus he never shows sloppiness.

He has piercing blue eyes, and if we do have a meal together, with other people, or alone, he discusses his son, what his wife makes him do around the house, his golf game, but mainly business.

He did not read my book. I don't know if this shows lack of curiosity or wisdom. I would say wisdom. Why should he know my inner life when he asks me continually to perform without emotion?

On the very rare occasions that travel makes it that we have a drink together, he says his marriage is difficult. "Whose isn't?" I reply. He makes it clear, though he is steadfast. The one trait a woman cannot resist.

He is always polite with me, rarely impatient. This is the gift of love he gives me.

I am no longer young, and why I would want to engage in a sexual language with him is odd. I know he looks at younger women. He may see me as a woman who was once attractive, or he may find me attractive. I want to know.

My being tries to draw him toward me. As if in challenge. He remains immutable, and this I find marvelous. The world feels fixed, has longevity.

The world is thus not victim to my misguided machinations. How many of my own ploys have ruined what is right for me. The boss does not allow this. For me or him. I can keep working with integrity.

Some people see this as cold. Indeed he is. His coldness saves us.

The boss never thinks of me. When he changes my office, he does not bother to tell me. He forewarns the man I am to change with. He apologizes to him. He does not even consider me.

Is this to do with my lower ranking as a female? Undoubtedly. This must be why his marriage is not good. He does not consider her either. He is in a man's world. I am hurt, but I do not show it, pretending I am like any man in service, while crossing and uncrossing my legs.

Why is it that women are attracted to their bosses? Is it as simple as the fact that we are in their care? They make the decisions that allow us to eat and to live. Right there, we are in a sexual situation.

My lover, being emotional, is the type of man who would talk to anyone sitting across from him about anything. He is always divining. He is a strategist and hopes to control people by what they reveal. My boss controls them by what he does not reveal.

My lover asks questions persistently, and the person sitting with him feels honored to be so interesting. My boss asks nothing, and the person begins talking in order to seem interesting.

My boss looks at my legs when I am in a meeting with him. Or my breasts. Just a quick look. A power move. He takes me. He acts as if he does not want me, and he takes me.

This behavior infuriates the feminist in me. But he does it so imperceptibly that no one could attack. One almost feels it was imagined. So I look for the connection. For any connection.

It is my job to be pleasant with him. Present the questions I have for him in a pleasant fashion. This is a sexual fawning in itself, but it is also part of my job.

The president's secretary just calls me and says, "You seem very down. You and the president both seem very down today. Did you two break up last night?" she jokes.

In my sadness she alludes to, I take sustenance in words. He has flow charts and monthly earnings to focus on.

When she tells me he is down, I am not surprised. I know he is an introvert, like me, and thus inside he rages emotion. He sublimates. And, in his earnings charts, forgets.

But would not anyone be down, corralled into an office daily? There is always the theatre in offices to entertain oneself, but a president is not privy to the on-stage and off-stage performances. Everything is made smooth for him when presented to him in his office.

Perhaps he enjoys my meetings because my sexual feeling is jagged, and, for that moment, we are human. Professional expectations are lowered.

Of course, what I really want is to be his second wife. I imagine I want this man, busy working his way up the corporate ladder and whose constancy is not to be even wondered at. I imagine he will bring order to my emotions.

The lonely erotic fire of the unattainable.

DOUBT IN WORK

It is very daunting for me to think anything I do is of any value. That is because I have read writers who are so much better than I, have worked with people who are far more intelligent than I.

I rely on my lover to say, "No, your work is good." "Is it?"

I ask, incredulous like a child.

I don't golf, play tennis, garden. My life is only the PC keyboard and books. Walks up and down Second Avenue. The rest of the time worrying about making money. But this small world has infinite space. A golf course in its manicured agenda smothers me.

FALLING IN LOVE WITH WORK

In the case of day jobs, one falls in love with the regularity of seeing the same people. Their consistency in being who you think they are. You go home with your image of them.

There's the incredible surprise when what you skittishly put together actually comes out as polished work.

You are not alone in working by the seat of your pants. Everyone else is doing it.

Finding out that occasionally you perceive originally, add value, as they say. The shock of it.

The flashes of ideas. Those ideas stand as themselves. They are things in themselves. Your offspring.

One rails against the strain, the pressure. But its chaos and demands force a focused energy that purifies one, as music does, as love can.

There's the pinch of working with people as family. In both places you make do, cleverly.

Friends call me who have the financial luxury to enable them to only make art. They are incensed when they have to do anything distracting. Their banking, for instance. The selling of their house. I am quiet, as I listen to them, for interruption is my life. I write in airports, at parties, in cars. George Sand got up from making love with Chopin to do her work.

You have to.

Then there's falling in love with the work of love. That is harder. Working alone is a passion I can control. The work of love is yielding to another.

The creative work is yielding to oneself. Why artists are called narcissistic.

The price for this life of creativity is financial insecurity. Often years go by where I lose money. But the gold I go for, the only one I respect, is the richness of freedom. I eschew security for the existential joy of freedom.

The novelist is the freest person, a novelist tells me. You find freedom in writing about traps.

That is why you love the man who loves you to do your work.

Work is action, opposing melancholy. Even the forgetting of yourself that takes place with work is wholesome.

Workaholism is a whole different thing, not always to be criticized. If the person was creating a vaccine, everyone would applaud him. If he is doing only his own work, people say it is an addiction.

Who was it that said, because he was lazy, he worked all the time. I agree.

I sit on a roadside in the sun to write my few pages. I am the happiest person alive, as Henry Miller said.

I have forged a life where I own nothing. My time is never taken up with dishes and mowing lawns. I admire those who do that, and even enjoy their generosity when they invite me to share in their home. It is their passion and I admire it. All I can give back is my conviction.

My conviction. The word they use when they sentence someone to prison. My sentence is my life.

A man works to "get" a woman. He works for her even when he wins her. You work at your relationship. You go to work every day. Recovering people speak of working their program. All of this is synonymous with pleasure.

We all muse about the freedom of not working. But none of us mean it. Even the children of wealth wish to be productive.

We should only do work we love. The healthiest of us love whatever work we do.

The pleasure is in giving oneself up, for whatever work it is.

It is work, the most terrible work, to be separated from whom and what we love. Why prison is a punishment. The work there is patience. The same is needed in waiting for work or for your beloved.

EXPERIMENT IN WORK

Sometimes it is experimental just to say what you truly believe.

When I work to please others, the result often is mediocre. When I take a chance and express myself, the work has a chance of standing out. At least.

Employers do want our minds and what is in them. They just want us to deliver our ideas in a way that is collaborative and not upsetting.

Using one's intelligence at work is usually experimental. Work gets slogged down by a compendium of collective doubts. Things only move when someone is affirmative.

It is experimental not to take work as everything.

Some people cannot help but want to do something different. No matter what they are told, no matter how much their superiors or editors want something seen before, some people approach a project with how can it be done differently. These people fail most of the time, and occasionally come up with rare flowers.

People who don't experiment at all with their lives, or who hold a job that does not inspire them, or who live with a spouse who does not inspire them, they experiment with nonexistence.

A single fifty-eight-year-old man returns yesterday from Puerto Rico, where he went to visit his aunts and uncles whom he never met. They are people in their seventies and eighties. He is experimenting with family.

A woman I know was an exotic dancer. Guliani closed down her places of employment. Plus, she is in her mid-forties, and although she still could dance, she perhaps would not make the money of a younger woman. She had never worked in a "straight" environment, where sex was not the tender. Now she works as a waitress in a cafe, walks dogs for money, and goes to school. She occasionally has sex for money. She experiments with independence.

A friend had too much imagination, too much desire. It bedeviled her. So she married a man with money and took a job on Wall Street, even though she has no interest in the stock market. By taking on such a prosaic life, she experimented with balance.

A friend lies about her age and spends her time studying new advances in plastic surgery. She has never worked but adopted a son so as to have some activity other than being bored by her husband. She goes to the gym, she travels, she fights with her husband, she raises her son. She is experimenting in doing it her way.

A woman had a powerful job and got meningitis. She now is a receptionist. She is happy.

A man tells me he is so busy with his demanding freelance that he gets up at three in the morning to work. I believe him, but I also know he fritters his time. He, like many men, likes the feel of the gun.

A highly successful friend was too critical for any man. One day she met a man for whom she suspended her critical judgement. They are getting married. She may stop working. She is experimenting with happiness.

I say that I would like to be supported, not wake up to having to "perform." Perhaps why I have no interest in performing in bed. I perform daily out of bed. My experiment would be in being kind to myself.

A lawyer begins writing vignettes from his experiences in small claims court. At first, all he could think of was making a deal with an agent. Of course, he was not made much of, along with the rest of the creative people. Now, he says he loves the writing itself. He is experimenting in being an artist.

"It was only later that I discovered that rebellion
Is a form of love."

—Paul Metcalf

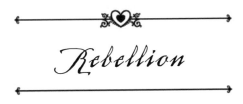

Rebellion

SELF-SABOTAGE

I have been enraged of late at the people in my life who did not encourage me. It was bad enough all the rejections, but on top of this I had to withstand others' lack of confidence in me, their mockery. In other words, I had to believe in myself by myself. Not an unusual situation for artists, but still bruising and painful.

My phone rings constantly when I am busy. This time it's a woman bored at home, sick. She is going through her phone book. "Reaching out," she calls it.

The real evil in seductiveness is not its Jezebel-like power, but how it attracts people into your life who waste your time.

The phone an assault weapon.

If it isn't a man I am ambivalent about, then it is a friend, a guest, a relative I become ambivalent about, all the while spending time with them.

A man calls me today "a free spirit but a limited one." Aren't we all?

A former boyfriend, when he was young, edited the college newspaper, won all the girls. He had energy and force. But he has spent the last thirty years smoking marijuana. He tells me his twenty-five-year marriage is boring, as is his job. He half-heartedly writes but makes no effort toward the discomfort of rising above mediocrity. He has smoked away his eros.

I had dinner last night with two friends from my long-distance past whom I have not seen in thirty years. One had his inquisitive and anxious ten-year-old son with him. Adult conversation happened in furtive looks and innuendo and responses to the son's questions. None of the adults connected. Only the son with his father.

I talk with a friend about the vagaries of making money. The ultimate sabotage to peace of mind. She is way behind on her rent. We discuss that making money is fundamental. Incredibly fundamental. You have to be willing to give up your time or your refinement to do it.

My broke friend sabotaged herself by not telling anyone of her dilemma. We all suffer from difficulties. But to wait until they are cataclysmic is sometimes an aggressive act of hostility to those around you.

We can fool no one. We are human, all too human, as Friedrich says.

The ultimate sabotage is holding onto the patterns that are the most chaotic. Funny how we cling to them. Let me go down on my ship.

DISTRACTIONS

The telephone as immediate distraction. Pick it up rather than sit through.

Listening to material I would have thrown in the garbage if handed to me in a book.

Worrying. Over this man, that man. This job firing me. This piece of copy sent. This possibility of my being dismissed, made useless, rendered invisible. Worrying that I will be abandoned.

Control by worrying.

I distract myself with male attention even if ill-fated. A married man. Or a mental hunchback. All for the warmth of the womb a man holds me in, for a little while.

Listening to people who are saying things you already know. It's not the news you want but the cooing, the mothering, reassuring, in that voice.

Wasting time pretending to reassure others, thus reassuring myself.

Wishing one was thinner, younger, more beautiful. If someone else cannot reject you, if someone else cannot abandon you, then by all means let's abandon ourselves.

Men whom you don't love but who amuse you. Who flatter you. Did I not say I distract myself with them? A way to pass time, but pleasurable.

It is a distraction to ask people for help in decisions. They do not know the real facts, so it is just a fobbing play at a momentary release from responsibility. Their answers only tell you of themselves.

Longing for my ex is a distraction from my loneliness.

Being unwilling to say, simply, "Help me." Complaining instead.

The distraction of the fantasies of happy endings. My books will sell. A man with money will arrive. I will be loved and cared for without much effort on my part. I will be loved and cared for in the way I want to be. Putting the nipple in the mouth.

PLEASING OTHER PEOPLE

I have made it my philosophy to give to people. But if I analyze it, I only do so to my comfort or pleasure. So, in a way, I am always only pleasing myself, bartering for my own affirmation.

The right love relationship is strengthened by pleasing one's daimon. The wrong love relationship feels diminished by one's daimon.

Sexually pleasing. I am not so advanced. I can only please by showing my pleasure. I am not aggressive in bed, as all men want, not a pleasure-giving machine. Inhibition? No. Laziness. There is so little extra, free time to give away.

My lover is giving. But I interpret it as control. So much of giving pleasure is control. Love me.

Often we are born into families of takers. When the taker parent dies, the desire to keep on giving to takers dies. One becomes self-protective, something trained givers must learn.

It has taken years for me to learn to spend time with people I actually like, not just people who dial my phone number in desperation.

Those people sound desperate from the first hello.

It has taken years to love those who are steady and manage their own lives successfully. I used to have the most compassion for the faltering. Now I believe the movement toward emotional and spiritual health is the only conversation worth having. The only conversation.

Sometimes you have to do with others what you do not want to. Sometimes you have to.

When you do, you grow, so usually this is a selfish act, too.

All acts are selfish. People say, "It is not all about me," but indeed it is.

THE IMPORTANCE OF THE ARGUMENT

I cannot stress how one must dissect everything said and seen and heard.

One must not swallow anything whole. One must check its texture throughout. And if any piece is not authentic, it must be regurgitated. Otherwise, too many years of your life can be lost.

If you commit to something, know it will require all, and be willing to give it. Otherwise, you will go nowhere.

Eventually the argument will tell you to love and be loved. To surrender. But if you have to get there by fighting every heart that demands, so be it.

I thought I was aggressing, but I was only defending.

I used to wonder, if I were all alone forever, what would I have to live for? And it seemed it would be music. In other words, the emotional infinite.

"In order to deceive melancholy, you must keep moving. Once you stop, it wakens, if in fact it has ever dozed off."

—E. M. Cioran

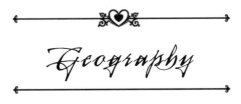

Geography

NEW YORK

My eternal passion for the streets. Coming up or into the skyline. Yes, the noise, the money, the rudeness. But the humanity, the theatre, the boundless opportunities for love. One has the illusion that one can be reborn.

One of the unspoken advantages of a harried life in New York is that I have no time for casual friends. Only the most intimate. Which means that things can only go deeper.

Overdrive. This is the age we live in, the city I live in.

It is the noise of defense that will drive me out of NYC. Car alarms, phones, police sirens, kids crashing bottles.

A man walks along the street wearing a plastic garbage bag as his winter jacket. This in the city about money.

Jackhammers again. The relief when they shut down. As when torture is reprieved.

In a small town, conversational exchanges are the beginning of something. In New York, they are moments that die. They are preparation for a quick and unexpected death.

There is art everywhere, in just the mosaic of how people are forced to live their lives.

A friend in the country looks out in solitude over his seacoast harbor every night. I have only recently realized I could not do that. I need the talking.

Tall slender woman in black and grey with shocking white blonde hair walking quickly. The epitome of New York.

Jackhammers again. I tell the man who sells me coffee. "The noise," I say. A young beautiful man. He grimaces in pain, too.

Men stride along looking like they would like to be taken in.

Women walk by in fur hats. This in the East Village where the last time a tie was seen, it was camp.

An usher from the local movie theatre dressed up in that black and white bojangles way hops down the street, bouncing an invisible basketball in front of him.

A man with AIDS blares his radio on the street. This while the New York police cadets walk by on their way to school.

A warm November day. It eases everyone's interior mechanisms. The lush life.

I see a man selling incense on the street. I know he is poor, so I buy some. What will $1.50 buy him in this city? However, my purchase will give him hope.

He looks through the incense bundles and says, "Serenity would be good for you."

I buy one leg of fried chicken from Kentucky Fried Chicken and eat it ravenously down the street.

A black man sauntering. A woman with her bulldog. A young woman in exercise clothes darting into a pastry shop.

At dinner we three New Yorkers speak fast, interrupt each other, compete with witticisms, theatricality. My lover, who lives in the country, is quiet, unable to hurl himself into the verbal fracas.

All the myriad distractions of the city converge into a directedness that is shaped without our shaping it.

When it was New York humid and hot, my ex complained incessantly. We would walk to Battery Park and stand by the Hudson River for some breeze. He would look longingly at the boats on the water. Perhaps seeing his future.

My ex loved the strong current, the impossible current, of the East River. For hours, he smoked cigarettes and studied it.

Thirty years ago my lover lived with a rock star in a very uptown apartment, complete with a large terrace and a view of Central Park. This is his knowledge of New York. Now he postpones living with me because the roughness of poverty in New York and the drive it necessitates are foreign to him.

TRAVEL

I travel six hours every week on business. I smoke cigarettes on the road, eat junk food, listen to music and fundamentalist stations that I would never normally listen to, and play out all kinds of scenarios. On the road, in the solitude of these hours, I always cry.

This morning I cried for a friend I am very close to, appreciating her. Usually I cry for my ex-husband. I am always, then, crying for home.

My last trip I cried when I saw a lit religious cross on a hill. This against the beauty of the sky. At that moment, it seemed clear there was a higher intelligence.

I love the houses I do not know, lives that seemingly go on in much better balance than my own. I imagine, driving by, all these lives as more settled than mine.

I drive myself, both literally and figuratively. I push on. I am Scott pushing on to the South Pole, for the pure rush of driving myself.

I cry at movies in airplanes, as I cry driving long distances in my car. Ergo when I am separated from my life, I experience the unequivocal pain of existential aloneness.

Some men I notice crave the existential aloneness of travel. But they become addicts—to alcohol, to power, to women, or to the comfort of work.

Conversely, I love the being trapped in my own world when I arrive in a new place. I am off my own turf and forced to go inward. I go into the quiet of my self. I become intimate with myself, as I am my only friend available.

The silence in travel is perfect for reading, as if the written word travels with you, through you.

I am not interested in "sights." To me every day is a "sight."

Therefore I love the suspension of travel but not the responsibilities of a new place.

My lover and I have not traveled much. Just getting to know each other became a fulsome journey.

Once again, it comes down to not being curious about the material world, but only the energy shift when I travel within my own consciousness.

I ask my lover, "Where did you go?" "To the cosmos," he says.

Continually, I say I want to get away. But I make no effort to do so. I passionately love my own streets, the man who sells me coffee, the young people who sell pastries and read books. The way the whole street strides. I get away on these streets when I am fully present.

My ex-husband used to fall in love with any woman who had a foreign accent. My lover said he saw a strikingly beautiful woman who is Russian. She speaks no English.

What are they longing for? To silence their limitations.

Beautiful views always heal. But they are all the same. A beautiful view tells us that the world is extraordinary. One need not travel for this.

The one place my ex and I did not fight was when we were in a car on the road. That was because I abdicated to him, and the journey.

As one overindulges one's eating habits when traveling alone, one imagines relaxing one's sexual habits. One feels one could easily fall into bed with a new person. A different form of travel.

I have always loved taking long road trips with lovers. The insularity in a car, a warm womb where communication is just as umbilical.

I have had thousands of sexual fantasies in cars and planes. Being found. Being taken.

Of course the advantage of travel is you get away from the sense that your life is of any importance. You see that lives are going on everywhere. There are other lexicons. You can raise or change the bar.

Another advantage is the slowing down of time. Without one's personal life to distract, time is slower. You live longer.

Traveling with no one to meet you is sad. Traveling with someone to meet you is limiting. Traveling with someone you know is redundant. You might as well have stayed home.

I am jealous of many things but almost never of people's trips. I am jealous of illuminating conversations, encouragement that others receive, unencumbered time.

I am, however, jealous of all the hotel rooms with unfamiliar men that I am not in a romantic clutch with.

Compared to New York, the rest of the world is on vacation.

THE OCEAN

The thunder of the sea. How many times it balanced me.

I love the sea and, like all of us, am umbilically tied to it, but I chose to live in the ocean of a city.

When I visit people who live on lakes or in the woods, I feel as if I am still in the city.

People by the sea live in active relationship with the colors, the tides. The instant changes in its moods. They sit on their porches and watch it, like one watches a lover's face.

My ex and I needed the sea to soothe us. We were both on fire, with grief, rage, need, and freedom, and only the sea was strong enough to douse us.

The sound of the gulls at 5 p.m., on the beach, when the light changed and the beach empties out, was always when I wanted to make love. I did do that when I was very young with lovers. However, when my ex and I lived together, he played baseball with friends at that hour, pointedly ignoring me.

My lover is not comfortable on a beach. To him, the beach is a backdrop. He wants me to talk to him or read to him. He does not go out to the actual sea of waves and tides. He wants to go out to sea in me.

The closest I get to the sea in daily life is music. I listen to music all day to keep the waves coming in.

I had a good sail today, my ex booms at me on the phone.

One is made beautiful in and by the sea. Why don't we all live there? Because the sea in one-self is what must be manifest.

I could not see living by the sea and not having a view. It would be like traveling centuries to Mecca and staying outside the town.

The rivers that border a city have none of the same power of the sea for me. I do not bother to walk to them for sustenance. Instead, I go up and down elevators, for conversation.

Sometimes my ex sends me photographs of the sea. He travels on it to Cuba, to Maine, to Key West. I look at the blue of the postcard, and I remember our love. How I plopped down beside him as we gazed out.

The sea is for those who have given up on people. And the intense friendships made there are those of people who do not want to go where something can be made with people.

The sea is whole in itself. Gods have been borne there. Great souls have died there. We were all once fish there. People who go to the sea to live are returning home.

We, who stay in the sea of activity, in cities, are struggling, struggling, with difficulty, to bring the human race further. Those, who stay by the sea, do not believe it can be done.

Life by the sea is for the discontented who crave contentment.

The city is for those optimists who will brave discontentment, in hopes they can fashion their lives into art or money. For those who live by the sea, there is nothing greater to fashion, except homage.

"If you are planning to write fiction, do not sit around too long trying to think up a good story. If you work hard, the story will come to life as you are writing it. Remember also that all decent fiction has the same inner story: the art of discovery."

—Robert Grudin

Art

ART VERSUS THE PC

The keys move quickly on a PC, so one has the illusion of productivity, no matter what one is writing. The image appears on the screen, as if you are already published. You can send it automatically to be read by someone, somewhere.

My ex could never learn a computer. He was shown many times but inherently refused. He liked to do things with his hands. He did not like speed. He did not like things to get ahead of him, the way typed words can.

If my ex and I played a computer game, he won on beginner. He is more linear, more logical. He won on intermediate. I won on advanced. Because of the speed.

I hear of love affairs on the Internet. People whom we lie about ourselves to (because that is all we can do).

Epistolary love affairs are nothing new, but e-affairs are another matter. This is the materialism of wanting someone and then dialing in for them and then presenting yourself in the words of a banner ad. "Where is the chemistry?" I ask a friend. Chemistry now is an anachronism. As if what people want to know about each other could be answered in a questionnaire. What hobbies you have, whether you prefer yellow or red. Through this, they think they can find love.

My lover must be fluent on the keyboard. He is fluent on the phone.

I am one of the outmoded people who do not trust the Internet because I know people's will to power. The Internet says come one, come all, which is the pioneer way, but all the cons and thugs of words are busy applying.

In my life, the phone still rings. People interrupt my life at the PC. The dog needs walking. My breasts need checking. Life demands. And like all people ensconced pristinely at the PC, the intrusion is painful.

The PC in truth, like all machinery, does not interest me. Don't be confused, I am as attached to it as the next person.

I switch on my laptop, as if it is my own heartbeat.

My laptop responds to me, is consistent. I can talk to it and it always listens. It is there for me without the vicissitudes of personality.

My lover says to me, "Well, the future is this software, that software. Novels will be read in palm pilots." I say to him, "You are reading the promotional writings for IPOs." I resist. I resist. Someone must insist on not rushing to the trough of commercialism.

The Chinese revolution had every citizen wearing the same clothes, in one style. The technology revolution will have us all reflecting the colors of PC screens.

PCs do not need care and feeding as a car does. Another reason we love them so. They perform for us tirelessly till they die of old age. The perfect mother.

One spends money on them as one does a lover. In other words, one spends too much. One spends more money than one expected to because they are as necessary as a lover.

I hardly use a pen except to make notations when I am driving or when noting matters related to phone calls. Those matters, if important, are transferred to the PC. My schedule is on the PC, and if the PC were to go down, so would my schedule. If the PC went down, I would have to be spontaneous. Let us hope I remember how.

CREATIVITY

One has to believe in oneself. Even in one's doubt. When one doesn't, one can't create.

If I am not being creative, I get creative with ways to destroy myself.

I see all relationships as transpiring in myth-form, not in so-called reality. Hence I can't maneuver myself through the dailiness of them.

I want to be loved and taken care of, but I live like a female warrior. I throw my javelin into the ring constantly to see if it will hurt. It hurts me.

Creativity comes out of pain for me. And sexual desire. I must have both operating at once. Which is not so hard to do.

Authenticity is original, pure glass.

Creativity as I have said is energy. One must get away from what dampens. Even depressives who are creative are energetic about their depression.

One has to feel that what one has to say is urgent. The rest is work.

Passion. One has to have passion for the geography in the story, the unyielding situation.

Writing is selection, nothing else. Selecting the right words, moods, settings, scenes.

What inspires imagination? Love. Any kind of love.

My lover wants to choose what he does, he says, by what is right for us as a couple. I abhor this. Those men who discovered countries, who made art, were not doing what was right for the couple.

But we are always talking about our own daimon.

Naguchi sculptures are not pretty, and because of that, I feel two things: grounded and earthy and safe, which then becomes sexual. I want to fuck Naguchi.

Writers make fun of their stand-in character in plays. The stand-in character for the writer is always weak. If a writer makes him out to be strong, he is a weak writer.

This morning I read that communing with God gives all the answers. I am sure this is true. And yet I so rarely do it. Which again shows me that I prefer the creative chaos to having God give me answers. The illusion of my free will.

My piano teacher gives voice to the notes. She sings a story to their sound. She hears breath. She says we have longer than we think to play them. There is more space in the moment than we think.

In my craving for what I call the intellectual life, I am simply craving more writing.

Sometimes I become totally enraged at my lover or, in the old days, with my ex-husband. I now wonder if I simply rage because I do not have the luxury of time to create.

ON WRITING

Writing is an experiment. People who like their own writing are suspect. They cannot withstand the anxiety of not knowing. They deem it good right away.

I should have been better.

Writing is the place I am brutally honest. Sometimes I don't push myself hard enough, and that work has to be deleted.

You have to cut out all the mediocrity. One should do the same in life.

It is deceptively easy to be brutally honest. In truth, it is most difficult. Most of us live easy lies, and this invades our writing.

For one who lives in her head, writing can be recriminating because one's head is not always that compelling.

Intelligent writers look out. Neurotic writers, like myself, look in. Some neurotic writers, like Kafka, can pull that off. But he was looking out, too.

Everyone but everyone thinks they are a writer. If they don't write, it is because they chose not to be a writer. Not because being a writer did not choose them.

I am always uncomfortable around people who think highly of their work. Perhaps because I don't of mine and think perhaps these people do indeed know how to open the vein. Their self-confidence is an added weapon in their artistic arsenal.

Some people read to mine their own minds. And some writers write for that.

Some people say writing is not pleasure. I do not find this true because I am interested in the discovery. Some books are written on first draft and then refined. Others are written in drafts, and the gold, after much burnishing, makes itself apparent.

Books whose intention is symphonic are written in draft after draft. Books that are akin to songs are written in early drafts.

I am amazed at how many writers write a story and then proffer it out to everyone they know—old lovers, future lovers, restaurant maitre ds, their therapists. Performance art, in a way.

The plethora of books about writing. I never learned a thing that way. It is something I learned by doing and feeling.

More was learned from obsessions. With what haunted me.

Woolf said novels are unlived desires. Of this, I agree.

I believe if there were heaven here on earth, it would be, for me, writing.

My ex's anger extended to my writing. He said I loved writing more than I loved him. I didn't, but I knew it would be a more constant friend.

THE FUTURE OF FICTION

Most people no longer look to novels for insight into humanity. A woman who is debating infidelity need not look to *Madame Bovary* or *Anna Karenina*; she can talk to her analyst or turn on the television.

Books and stories often seem arbitrary because we have all been analyzed (or seen enough people affected by analysis) to know that life is even more complex than written stories reveal.

Fiction, in short, seems simplistic.

Of course, language can become an art form in itself. The ear becomes the source of pleasure, as with music.

While fiction can no longer offer paths to understanding life, more and more people are writing it. As someone told me, it takes no investment. You don't have to buy anything; you just sit down and write. It's easy, he told me.

But, indeed, more and more people are writing it, people without any interest in psychology, even, which makes for a disconnect. Editors are being inundated with work about situations that the writers are not even affected by.

There is nothing unspeakable since we are an age of confession, an age of mass information. TV shows try to outwit each other in discovering pockets of what is still unspeakable. Nothing shocks anymore, except perhaps goodness.

The rise of Christian and Jewish and other religious literature is trying to find out if it's in the avant garde. Because these are stories based on past notions, and made up of over-simplified plots where the good destroys the bad, these books cannot be true literature.

Now we must make it new, as Pound said, but also make it more relevant than the analyst's couch, the television interview.

No one likes to hear this except natural-born rebels, and true artists are by nature natural born rebels, if only in their work. Creativity depends on destructive power, and one must take all the pieces apart and put it together again.

In middle age, which I am in, we are a little gun-shy. We have suffered so to attain a modicum of continuity.

But the artist must win out over the bourgeois. Perhaps why so many artists like to be with the young. They still question form.

My ex doesn't read fiction. He finds no use for it. Being so emotional, he distrusts emotion.

He wants the solidity of fact, the solidity of history. Fiction, to him, is like dating a neurotic woman.

My landlord never reads fiction. His own life overwhelms him enough.

"There is something of the charlatan in anyone who triumphs in any realm whatever."
—E. M. Cioran

Against

Society

COMMERCIALISM

No one, now, even if they're clamoring after it, trusts the buzz. We all know what it is: a buzz.

Since psychology and psychoanalysis have replaced novels as sources of guidance and wisdom, novels primarily entertain.

Subtlety is gone. Editors ask the person truly traumatized and thus living a life in indirection to plug on the yellow star. Make it big like a screen.

Nobody wants to watch real pain, such as watching a lover brush his lover's teeth because his lover is too sick to hold his toothbrush. Give me, instead, death by computerized giant waves.

Packages and pictures: can we sell this book with this DVD of this movie? Can we overexpose ourselves? Overfeed the consumers until their senses are dulled. They'll become addicted to overexposure and we'll stay in business.

When I see old people, what strikes me is how little stimulation they need. In our "full-powered time," we grab everything, keeping ourselves from ourselves.

Friends are those who separate the chaff for us.

Commercialism as king will die because we can't see beauty for the noise. But the soul craves beauty, so eventually it is beauty that will win out.

Cities of commerce, like New York, attract the artists but not so much the audience they need. The art world is confused. Here we gave you all this, and the consumer says, It's too much. Everyone must sort themselves out from the tumult.

The line drawing comes back, the unexpected simple story gains an audience.

Unaware that art has failed them by selling out, some people turn to new age religion to satisfy their craving for beauty. This is a serious failure of art.

Artists like to blame the commercial handlers, but we should blame ourselves for playing into them.

It is natural to want to blaze before we die. Shall it be a flashy glitter or a deep ember? The deep ember of course requires the long patience, and no one may see it.

Travel, reading, dressing, aging now have all become matters of commercialism. Huxley said the ad writer would be read by millions. Whatever we discover of use soon gets tarted up and presented as something extraordinary. We are to think only in superlatives.

We have dismissed the ordinary.

MONEY

I have reached the advanced age where men lure me not with passionate kisses and rides in convertibles but with promises of money and security.

Money is a foreign substance to me. I do not make efforts to attract or save it. I wait for money and myself to surprisingly collide.

Part of the magic of my life is the waiting for money to come in some unforeseen way. I will not be shackled to what it takes to have it. This I wrongly deem as some kind of purity.

My fate is such that no money came through relatives or marriage. This has often been interpreted by my psyche as my being undeserving.

When people speak of money, I am bored, as people are when a subject they do not understand or care about is discussed. This has made me a boring dinner companion to many men.

Most of my friends have money. They have mastered its mysteries. I am the child with them. I am ashamed of this, although I shyly proffer the gold of my freedom.

As when I was young, wealth was sandals with my toes shining through. The sun hitting any cranny. Unexpected smiles, unexpected connections. Music.

For some unknown reason, I expect men to understand the vagaries of money although I have often chosen men who don't. I expect them to understand money as men expect women to understand mothering. Intuitively.

My father raised me to be saved. It was his own longing to be saved that he imparted to me.

He fouled this plan by teaching me only one thing: defiance. He taught by example. This defiance has sabotaged any possible chance of my being saved. I kick the savior to show my independence.

I cannot save. Saving means I will need in the future. I defy my aging by not saving.

Friends tell me money is not mysterious. You are intelligent, they say, you can master it. But they forget that my blindness is my insistence that the prince will arrive. In fact, he must. I will wait faithfully.

I will not let the fairy tale down. Someone must believe.

All my life I have spent more than I earned. Spent it on friends, spent it on myself. I was not materialistic, indeed always lived with few possessions, but I was quick to give a present, quick to give a present to myself. Quick to pick up the check. I never saw it as money being spent. Just an energy exchange.

Friends know me as a soft touch. They borrow money from me that they don't repay. But really that says more about the friend than myself.

People who live within a budget are Chinese mathematicians to me.

I see many people who live on far less than I do. I imagine it as self-containment.

Being a woman is an enormous expense. The clothes, the face creams, the hair, the fingernails. Some women eschew all that. But if you are in a fairy tale, you must look like a princess.

I see photos of myself when I was a young woman. I had no money at all then. However, I see no difference in my dress or bearing than I do now in my expensive clothes and expensive makeup.

The vulnerability of not having money makes you one with all people. Another way one fights isolation.

My lover feels that our problems can be solved by his earning more money. It will help, but it won't ease any loneliness.

ON NOT HAVING CHILDREN

It seemed that I was heeding Beckett's words, "the dedication, the single-mindedness necessary to realize, against all odds, one's artistic potential." I told myself I cannot divert in any way. I forgot how I frittered time on so many other activities that were far less enriching than having a child.

I doubted my patience.

I doubted my envy. My child would get so much more love than I did, even from me, and I would be abandoned again.

This is how I thought.

I espoused Cioran's words: "Those children I never wanted to have—if only they knew what happiness they owe me!"

None of my best friends have children. And if they do, the children are adopted.

I adopted forlorn and lost men, as lovers.

I stare at children as if they are extra-terrestrial beings. I am a bit frightened of their beauty and spiritedness. They are unfettered. I want to be them.

But, like Cioran, am too sad.

Beethoven, Nietzsche, Beckett, Woolf, so many did not have children. Of course they may have wanted them, and like me, fearful circumstances prevailed, thus they were left with work. I am not equating their illustriousness to my own garbled efforts. Many people have not had children. I note these geniuses because all of them were depressed, although, at times, jubilant in their work.

But their sadness, their sadness would not let them propagate.

A woman without children is considered unnatural, unfulfilled. This is untrue. It is true her animus is stronger. She lives parts of a man's life by not fostering another's. She has time to conquer the external world. A childless woman's hopes lie solely in herself, not in her progeny.

Having hope solely in oneself is a terrible burden and responsibility. Many women give themselves the backup of having children.

The childless woman is to be judged (by herself) critically.

Men see you as a woman who could not be had. A childless woman is no one's vessel but her own. Too often, a vessel of sadness, but her own vessel nonetheless.

There is a special aloneness of the childless woman. She risks dying alone, dependent on the kindness of strangers, the all-time most evocative of phrases. But a childless woman has already wagered that everyone dies alone.

ON FAME OR LACK OF IT

When you're young, you want it as a vehicle for revenge against all the past hurts. Now they'll know who I am.

When you're older, you know it will make little difference, or perhaps only bring new pains of being misunderstood. In essence, fame has all the same pitfalls as any relationship. It does not live up to its hopes, and it brings with it its own steady flood of limitations and embarrassments.

People project onto you constantly. You are a special being. They look to you to find out what it takes to have done whatever you are famous for. You must have had a stronger finger from God. And perhaps the famous do. After all, they have unusual talent in some way, if only for understanding the media.

To be touched by God would be to have plentiful talent and beauty. The famous, thus, give us a little preview of heaven. We will be this, and more.

But, in this life, the famous are not yet with God, and hence to know the famous is to know the club foot also.

To be a person whom fame never touches is another matter. One feels in some way as if one failed. One was not bright enough a light. Then it is to our friends we look for our mirror. To them, we must shine. And, for some, our families.

Some will tell you that they are famous. They are not.

Some eschew the light, mock it, and attract it nonetheless. Their mockery reflects everyone's desire for freedom from the desire for fame.

Beauty offers a transient fame. Yes, we all remember Monroe and Hayworth. But their beauty was also their generosity. That they smiled continually for us, continually made themselves up so we could enjoy their beauty, as they did. Here, look at me. Isn't it amazing? Let's share it and laugh at it and be amazed by it. Their generosity of spirit and humor matched their beauty. Plenty of even more beautiful people have never been seen or have been forgotten.

Some people immortalize their friends by giving them nicknames. Even on construction sites, laborers dub carpenters as "Words" or "The Lone Builder." These names create a legend.

One can seek out fame from the collective but never from individuals. That is a gift.

Fame, however, to the sensitive, hurts. As if the light shines too brightly. As if they know that the God who has given them talent does not want it displayed as newspaper material.

Advertising preys on all the clichés of fame. The smile. The tears. The aspirations. They make sure that when readers scan the ads, the images lull the readers into believing that, for that instant, they are near the light.

Some people become famous merely by their good works. They are not famous in *People Magazine* but with other seekers of God. They know they must give themselves away.

Now everything can be found on the Internet. You can make yourself famous on the net.

In this age of focusing on the famous, are we really exposing our need for signs of God? Our longing for fame is really a longing for the beauty and talents of heaven, a longing for the divine.

To children, animals are worthy of fame. They project all the goodness in their own hearts onto the animals. Intuitively, they know it is not so simple with humans.

PSYCHOANALYSIS

Psychoanalysts travel about as gunslingers, touched by their own kind of aura. After all, they are healers. Their words can shoot into the heart and transform.

I put analysis behind work. When there is too much work, I cannot fit it in. In other words, the objective saves.

I have seen psychoanalysis help and I have seen it not help people. It is not an antibiotic.

It is true that much of our mind is tortured, and, when it is, it is because what we feel is hidden.

I had a Freudian to begin with. They are clear. They believe in responsibility, they do not believe in happiness. They believe, however, you can get what you want. What you want won't make you happy, but you will be changed.

My Jungian analyst, when I come in with relationship problems, sees them as only problems in my relationship to myself.

I have friends who are in daily psychoanalysis and then in couple psychoanalysis. They are in their fifties and still amazed at their mothers. Their analysis works in that they make incremental changes toward commitment to each other or making money. Would they otherwise?

Many artists are suspicious that psychoanalysis will exorcise their demons and thus their material. Psychoanalysis can never exorcise the demons. The hurt always exists.

I found out through psychoanalysis that not everything was my fault.

I found out that most of what I think about my lover, I think about myself. The good and the bad.

I found out that I had been terribly hurt. Everyone finds that out.

I cannot go out with a man who is not psychoanalyzed. Some part of the conversation is stilted. The man is dealing with a patina of himself. And asking me to accept it.

What would be unleashed in me if there was no lover, no husband, no psychoanalyst? I would set out for Spain and bump into America, perhaps.

Couples therapy is wonderful. The truth comes out, the truth that is hidden behind smiles and sexuality. The truth of how you both are avoiding the truth.

There is a film called *Four Feathers* about four men who were cowards and had to lose their feathers (signs of cowardice) by acts of bravery. These four men went to war and rescued one another. If they had been in psychoanalysis, they would have talked forever about fearfulness on the couch.

My ex has grown in his sea town, on his boat alone, through his trips, his interests, without psychoanalysis. This tells me that psychoanalysis may not be necessary. He has not changed, but he has grown more intrinsically into himself.

Those who give emotions the lowest priority and those who give them all priority are prime candidates for psychoanalysis. That includes all of us some of the time.

Psychoanalysis tells those who are timid to listen to themselves. It tells those who are abrasive not to listen to themselves.

Perhaps psychoanalysis is purely to change the self, not to become the self.

New York, city of ambition, is all about how can I change myself: to be even more successful? More loved? More beautiful?

"It is not by genius, it is by suffering, by suffering only, that one ceases to be a marionette."

—E. M. Cioran

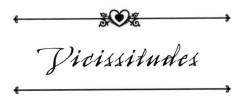

Vicissitudes

AGING

The older we are, the better we know how to love. We have had so much of ourselves that we can be less self-consumed, take a break from our careful watch. That is why love in later years is so passionate.

I know that biology has a powerful pull in sexuality, but I can no longer offer a lover his progeny. Now the pull must be in knowing, that I can truly know him.

I watch marriages fall apart in later life because one party in the marriage is hungry for truth. Duty is a challenge to the young, a false god to the old.

Working for someone else is less important to the aging. One answers in later life to one's own rhythms.

My ex has a young true love. She is obsessed with the perfection of her body, people tell me. This information has aged me.

My lover tells me that I am beautiful as I am. He wants to be with someone old, he tells me.

My friendships when young were endless discussions, trying to sort out our confusion and resentments and unconscious passions. Now we share our interests.

People are more patient as they age. We understand that we repeat our mistakes over and over. Nothing is cataclysmic. The tides keep coming in.

There is no greater pleasure than walking. To think that old age can take that away. But then I suppose there is pleasure in flying down the street in your wheelchair.

Why we cry when we watch a handicapped race: These people have found pleasure in whatever the circumstance of their lives. They affirm the resilience of the human spirit. We know we will need it more and more for ourselves as we age.

I worry that I cannot keep my lover in my thrall, now that my face is less pretty. I look at young women, and all of them are pretty. I cannot believe that my sexuality can reside in the force of my personality.

And yet, even though I am older, I become as a girl with my lover. I kiss him as we drive. I smile. Perhaps sexuality is in giving and being loved, not in smooth bare shoulders.

And yet some of me looks forward to the lack of preoccupation with the sexual theatre, and the compensating interest in art. But another part of me knows that the sexual theatre never really closes.

More and more when I read of men and women in love, the women are younger than me. No one falls hopelessly in love, in literature, with a woman in her fifties. And yet I see it all the time around me in life.

My lover tells me of sixty-year-old women he finds sexually attractive. He never tells me of young women he finds sexually attractive.

Now other women are referred to as the "pretty woman." Not myself.

Women in Europe are less anxious to hide their age. They sit at dinner with their glasses on, their fixed expressions. Sexuality for them is not about the puella.

A friend says to me, as the girl in me dies, fewer men who are boys will be attracted to me. Now it will be the men.

I am to go to my mother's hospital tomorrow. She is in the geriatric wing, where my brother says they are all waiting to die. Many of them, like my mother, have lost their minds. I hope I can be strong and loving and I can be clever enough not to wait to begin the life I want.

Is the life we are living ever the life we want?

We admire people who have insisted on their own lives, no matter at what selfish cost to others. We admire that they saw how finite it all is.

We spend our lives doing things we are not particularly interested in and then eventually tell ourselves we were interested in those things. In hindsight, those things define us to ourselves.

As an American, I look at my facial lines and think what can I do about it? What can I buy/spend money on to have them taken away, all the while knowing any solution is temporary. We bring consumerism even to this process.

To age without family or love is a cruel, cold journey. Some people, like myself, are foolish enough to insist on it, thinking that there is fresh information there. In remaining pure and unsullied. Perhaps wisdom can enter us more easily. We are freer for God.

We are the ones who would have gone to the Cross.

FINANCIAL STRUGGLE

People in the United States don't have the money or the assuredness of abundance we used to have. Doors are closing. We can't get jobs as quickly or as easily as before. We now have to be grateful for what we have.

It is a time of inner resources. The people with big hearts are ready.

Those who have lived close to the ground are the teachers.

We talk about the economy like it is an excuse for where we failed.

All of us who mocked capitalism suddenly are surprised by the way the center is not holding. Maybe we were right after all.

Americans are optimists. We can beat this. What is needed now are good ideas, not the belief that old systems will work. Good ideas. It is the creatives' time.

We don't need more efficiency, the promise of most goods over the past twenty years. We don't need more production horse races. We need steadiness. Our own, more than anything.

"The more perfect the artist the more completely separate in him will be the man who suffers and the mind which creates."

—T. S. Eliot

YOU ASKED WHAT HAPPENED WITH MY LOVER

Then, without asking me, I came home and he was there. Who is this stranger? This man watching golf, needing food, taking naps, talking about money. Who is this stranger?

I could not sleep. He was trying to fill the space of my imagination. With himself. I could not sleep, lying in the dark, recalling myself. Recalling the Other.

You must go back, I said. Go back to your town and build your life. I will be your lover, I will be your mistress, but I cannot be your meaning. Go back.

And he did. As my husband did.

And then I began searching, struggling, flirting, screaming, walking, listening, talking, listening, to get back to my work.

I chose loneliness again.

"Why is it that all men who have become outstanding in philosophy, statesmanship, poetry, and the arts are melancholic?"

—Aristotle

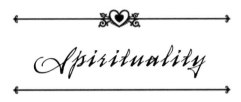

Spirituality

ARE WE ALONE?

My friend and I realized that, as of the year 2003, there were twenty-eight million menopausal women with economic power. We are a generation of women who broke out. For an instance, this piece of information explains why we are not with our first husbands.

Intimacy for me is being able to do my work while being involved with someone. I measure it by how well I can be on my own with someone.

Why do friends tell me I have French sensibility? It is because I dissect love with seven toothcombs.

My lover suggested that we get married but not live in the same state. My heart flowed open at the idea, but it was not the marriage part of the sentence.

I see that when I cry in grief and mourning, I am strengthened right after. Nothing terrible happens.

A woman discussing her every feeling minutely. This woman mines her behavior in the hopes of discovering the secret of a perfect outcome.

My lover tried to tell me that my home should be with him. That he would be the home. I tell myself I am too old for that. I am my own home.

The writer, Olive Shreiner's, ideas were strong and half baked. She was always leaving some man, even a husband, to be on her own. She called these leavings "attending to her health problems."

In Olive Shreiner's time, people communicated by letter. Now we have the phone or email. There is no lapse between words. We give in to gut reaction, not the pondering of the mind.

The head/rationality, in our time, has become a pariah. Everyone wants to trust only their emotions. People think it was ideas alone that caused mayhem. But it was emotion, without worthy ideas, to guide them.

I fear more than anything my lover's sentimentality.

WHAT IS IT WE LOVE?

Any focus, on one's lover or on one's work, is prayer.

My ex, after we split, first put his love into building his boat, into the sea, and then into yoga. He was diligent about all three, immersing himself so as to forget me. And then he met a woman who could give him what he wanted.

I run into friends in the hallway, and we share a cigarette and reflect on all that has come true that we always knew was true. How long our own inner lives take to manifest is solely dependent on how much of our own anxiety we are ready to give up.

This morning silence is exquisite. A minister says if a minister repeats, he is either not prepared or emphatic. Of this love of silence, I am emphatic.

Summer so beautiful. Especially as it now ends. My friend invites me to dine outside. "Yes," I say, "let's do it, especially since there are only three weeks left." "Oh no," she says, "there will be Indian summer."

Over and over my lover tells me he loves me. Still, even after I have banished him physically. But he insists on telling me how much he loves me. He becomes transcendent, is made whole, excites himself, purifies himself with the frenzied ecstasy of outpouring his love.

When one is striving, one heeds every message as a sign to keep striving. One relates to all that strives. When one achieves a moment of success, one must still strive. If one relaxes, all may be lost.

Therapy tries to uncover the reasons for our malfunctions. Religion simply says there is something bigger than the malfunction. In other words, rise above it.

I read a bit of the New Testament, and I learn that if you ask and believe, you shall receive. I have to say, that in my experience, this has been true.

This morning, as I work for the engineers, as I walk a hot road in Houston, I decide I should move to Somalia and help refugees. I must do something meaningful. Then I flash forward to my ex hearing how I have been shot rescuing children. The children are saved and I am dead. I even withstand torture. Clearly, I want to get rid of myself, for his sake.

It is difficult to pray because to pray you must commit to what it is you want and need. You must be humble enough to ask. You must both limit yourself and enlarge yourself. What you are given back is the truth.

Christ knew what his fate was. Redemption only after a hard time.

To live is to be constantly humiliated by one's character flaws.

A life of total humiliation in exchange for the gift of sensitivity.

I have been checkmated in life, given no money, family, or home, so as to stay close to the spiritual, to the marginal.

What is charisma? Excitement. Even if it's internal.

Dogs wait patiently for their masters. They make themselves comfortable, watching the door. Dogs love, they simply love. They are devoted perfection.

Children point to the dogs, perhaps sensing this perfection.

I smoked a cigar with the engineers last night. To join in communion with them.

My lover has no books around his apartment except mine. That tells the whole story. Its attractions and its repulsions.

Strength against fear comes for some from the words of the Bible. Knowing God will deliver if you trust. Those Black women reading the Bible could frighten Malcolm X with their lack of fear. And they did.

"You look sorrowful," a friend says.

I hear on the radio on one of those fundamentalist programs, I hear that one must give one's loss to God. Listening, I become empowered to let my ex, whom I love, go. That he does not belong to me, as I like to believe. He belongs to his own life of love.

The fact is we are caught in a strange situation. We do not know what is next for us, what joys, we do not know what joys are before us, but we know how adept or strangled we are at allowing them.

I spend more than twenty-four hours in complete solitude. With short stories. With food. With people I do not know around me. I sit by the Rhine in the sun and read. I sleep deeply from jet lag in a hotel bed. I am in full sensual communion with loneliness.

DISCERNMENT

When a man talks about sex during dinner, using evolutionary biology as a subject, getting to how a man leaves his sperm everywhere, you must be discerning.

When he says, "You are difficult."

"How?" you ask.

"Well," he says, defeated, "I hit on you and nothing came of it."

When he takes your hand in the movies, but he has a girlfriend he has talked about, and you have a boyfriend you have equivocated about, then you must be discerning.

When a man sends you a poem he has written and the writing is full of cliches, be discerning.

When your lover thinks that your own marriage together will not be torture, be discerning.

When a person you work with wants to engage you in snickering at others. He thinks this sniping is bonding, and your stomach becomes revolted; be discerning.

When your friends don't encourage you to wait for an intelligent man, be discerning.

When a friend calls upset because her roof falls in, but she is giggling. And she wants your ex-husband's phone number.

Men who read newspapers are discerning. They are willing, willing to navigate the world as it is.

When a friend has no time to talk to you, be discerning.

When a friend gives you the temperature of her feelings, even on the answering machine, thinking that this is interesting, be discerning.

So many things conspire against discernment. One's sexual desire. One's need for love. One's need to be soothed. Any devil will do.

Silence is discerning.

Free time is discerning. There is no lying to oneself when one is not busy.

Most men would like to abdicate discernment and let the woman decide for them.

Children are naturally discerning, emotionally.

Doctors, one finds out to one's chagrin, are not discerning. They are only busy.

I all too often interpret a person's silence as an act against me. This is not discerning.

Laughter is relaxed discernment.

Making love with someone one enjoys making love with is discernment.

Allowing oneself pleasure, of a lunch in the sun, dim sum that one enjoys, doing something new, is discernment.

ON DEEPENING

Sleeping alone and letting my dreams and feelings take over.

Even the waiting through winter, the agony of it, for the sun, is a kind of happiness.

To be alone is not defeat, not error. It is a relationship, also. Complex, fickle, emotional. A friendship with someone of identical interests.

To be able to listen. To shut the hell up and listen. There are always doors trying to open.

On being still enough to make love. Not to make love out of anxiety. Anxious love is rough, even hurts. To be still enough to let someone in.

To give love over and over and over. But much harder, to stand still when you are receiving it.

God. To find out. To read. To listen. To be open. The soul does hunger, that we know. So what are we saying when we say God?

The Fundamentalists insist it is Jesus. A phantasmagorical story that is hard to accept. And yet it has lasted for so many centuries. One story that took. People want to devote themselves to a savior. At its core, humanity is female and wants to surrender.

Music uplifts. It is a mood changer, like alcohol. Sometimes we need to be uplifted. But silence deepens.

My lover is Christ-like to me in that he only wants to give me love. He wants me to devote myself to him, have faith in him, and surrender to him. Is he usurping God's place? Is this pathology or is God at work?

To be content with my lover's calls. To be content with the way he says, "What, honey?"

HUMOR

Some people laugh at an unusual word placed in a sentence.

A word they do not often use. Like the word "klink."

Some people think it is funny to put other people down.

It isn't. Only the audacity of it is faintly attractive.

Some people like to laugh at themselves. This is attractive only briefly. After a while, one knows it is a defense.

When people are honest, it almost seems funny. We are so unused to it. Most people have to couch their honesty in a type of humor, so people will find it palatable.

I am a person who is not that interested in jokes. I'm surprised when they're funny. But mostly I feel confined by the proscribed nature of jokes. I like improvisation.

Wit. The wine of minds.

Some people can flirt and make it funny. This is creative. Their performance is in the moment, not from a seductive arsenal from which they pull material.

Humorists are gods. I knew one who sat down with two stuffed animals and began a long, unpredictable conversation. He wondered what the horse whisperer was saying to the horse. He said it was, "Shut up and listen."

People who don't work for a living have no idea of how much humor you need just to stay above water.

Dogs have wonderful humor. They don't know they have it, but they enjoy you playing with their jokes.

Some people dress humorously. The unexpected tie. The strange bracelet. They are telling you that all does not appear as it seems.

When people are sexually attracted, they tend to joke. It is a way of fawning.

Sometimes it is also a way of just amusing oneself when one is bored.

With people you are not interested in, you just go bang bang bang through the work to get the work done. Don't bother with the niceties. On the other hand, with people you enjoy, you can't help quipping, laughing, joking. Humor prolongs the experience.

HUNCHES

The only difficulty I can see is that one doesn't listen to one's hunches. They seem guileless.

I have known everything that happened to me before it happened. I just never heeded it.

My hunch is that many of my women friends who complain about their spouses complain to feel like they have the upper hand.

All artists rage to be validated. I am not chastising, only stating.

Some people make telephone calls, on and on, as if it is work. Instigating a call makes them feel important.

My lover swept me away on the rip tide of his need. I could not help but be swept. But finally I came into the shore of myself.

Mornings alone in my apartment are the height of sensuality. Women writers everywhere have drunk in this sensuality as more powerful than being with any lover.

Catherine Deneuve now. Her beautiful features worn by feeling. She is no longer an icon of cold perfection, now an icon of emotion. Lines around the eyes, paleness, a loss of a waist. No one is to be ashamed.

SOLITUDE

Solitary mornings are extraordinary. Silence. The pleasure of eating alone. The life of dreams folds into the day.

Walking in silence. In relationship to all.

How can one person (a beloved) compete with the solitary pleasure of being in conjunction to the universe?

Old people move toward that silence. As they age, they move away from the conundrum of daily life and move into the solitary roar of the eternal.

I was always frightened of solitude, knowing that eventually I would end up there. Knowing it would be intrinsic to me. I knew I would belong to it. We all do, if we allow it.

People who have been alone for many years are seen as odd, maladjusted. Perhaps it is quite the opposite.

It is not just that in solitude you can control your environs. Because you can't. In solitude, your emotions run wild and take you traveling.

I tell my ex that I have fewer and fewer friends. All my friends have merged with their men. I have merged with solitude. He says, "Sounds more writerly."

The beats were great socializers. Or is that myth? Every writer feels profoundly alone except when writing.

Solitude frightened me. Now I fear not having enough.

A friend tells me he prayed to be delivered of the desire for women. His prayer was answered, and he is happy in his solitude. He loves everyone, and no one clamors for his single-minded attention.

A woman I know moved to the country by herself. The news, she says, is she got a new kitten.

Another friend moved to the country for the solitude. Her news? She met the man she plans to marry.

The commitment to solitude, in other words, brings unexpected gifts.

Evenings are the hardest. The times you wish you had someone to talk to. The hours you worry most. If only . . . but they pass, and the morning brings its recurring gift of promise.

There are times one looks beautiful, but only for oneself. That seems wrong. It's not.

One reason people stay alone is for possibility. Some people see that as wanting a continual fix. But I see it more as wanting the freedom to keep growing beyond oneself.

Intelligent people are always chafing within their marriage. This conversation again? they wonder. But in solitude, one has the same conversations over and over again, also. However, there is hope of a different outcome.

When one is alone, one is more creative. Even just about mundane duties, because one is free to be putting ideas together, free to realize them.

One's passions are living entities. They take over. A state of ecstasy.

A couple I know have many children. They write. They work. They have many houses. I imagine they find the rewards of solitude in walks with their dog, being out in their boat, holding each other in bed.

Some marriages change with age, and the husband gets his own house, the wife keeps hers. They are not separated, but they have arrived at the point where everyone needs more of a relationship to self. A healthy marriage, as Rilke said, encourages this.

Most marriages, as I have said, between artistic people go away and toward.

Theatrical and vocal music distract from inner solitude, but classical music and jazz return you to it.

In solitude, the sun and moon become one's associates.

Sleeping alone is important to imagination. I used to get up, when I was married, to sleep on the couch so I could dream more openly.

"Committed to the future—even if that only means *se preparer a bien mourir.*"

—Dag Hammarskjold

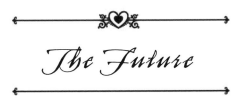

The Future

ACCEPTING MISTAKES

That I will not always know what is driving me, no matter how much analysis I have.

That friends and lovers will change because I have changed. That, in the transition, there will be confusion.

It will be a mistake to forget death but not to forget my anxiety.

I make the mistake of total distraction in this the city of distractions.

The mistake would be to take my silly daily perturbations and make them more important than enjoying my life.

My mistake would be thinking time is infinite.

My face tells me that time is not infinite. One must do what one intrinsically believes is important now. There is no time to do otherwise.

The mistake is to think one is powerless.

ON STARTING OVER

One has to, in a way, look brightly to the future. One has to, most difficult of all, believe in a happy ending. This time.

Or one can just let life happen. That is a way, too.

One has to know one cannot see the road before us anyway. We have no idea what we look like, what impact our work has, what our love is made of. One can only take care of one's body, work hard at one's vocations and avocations, and love the people we are busy loving.

If we do not know whom we love, we must be loving all the time to everyone.

Why optimists love the mornings: Today I will do something well. Something that is good. I will make something. I will come through for the person I love.

Sometimes optimism fails. One believes that no new history can be written. One refuses to start over.

"Starting over" is another expression for investing in the present. I will love again.

Intelligently, one should weed out what is not good about one's life and replace it with what feeds you. To do this, one has to take time away from one's routines to discover what feeds you.

I drive a lot for my work. It is during those times I look at the weeds in my life and think about what can be done to improve my lot.

Starting over requires action. Fear defies action. Things are never as impossible as one thinks. One should only forge on.

It is difficult for me to start over because I am so aware of the continuity of my defects. And yet these same defects continually force me to have to start over.

If it makes you uncomfortable, it might be calling you.

In other words, you have to be willing for life to be better than you imagine. Your openness encourages the imagination of others to augment yours.

Sometimes letting people help you is a form of starting over. To keep your mouth shut and let people tell you what they see, how they would do it. Then you may get a sense of a new world.

My ex once yelled at me that I had forced him to date. I had not done what he wanted, and now he had to start over. Now he is happier than when he was with me.

If you need to start over, it is because your world has atrophied.

After a divorce is an ideal time. You are young again. Your skin may not be a young woman's, your body not as alluring, but your nature is as vulnerable, your hopes as tenuous.

Fate becomes your lover.

Each moment I intend to start over, my mind slogs through all its rubbish, and each moment I have to free myself of it.

It is difficult to start over with friends from the past. They want to hold you to how they knew you. They are not so willing to watch you jump to the next island. They would have to explore the nature of starting over themselves. They are both envious of your opportunity, your energy, and aware that you may be going nowhere.

All of us have trouble with the futility of our attempts. No one is happy, except briefly. Part of starting over is to accept that.

DOING SOMETHING NEW

First, you grieve that one thing is ended. You really grieve. Then you turn around and you say, What if?

If you gravitate toward it, you move.

You try not to worry.

You believe.

DEATH BED

What will be important? My lover who will have spent years with me. Whoever he is.

Books. How they made me happy. And when someone understood my story, it was as if the story had its own life.

Sitting on the beach at Coney Island with a close friend who had been there sixty-five years ago as a child.

The times I laughed will not seem that important. Or cried. Just the times I gave myself.

Knocking at the door of God. I will think I should have knocked harder. It would have been another complex relationship.

The faces from work will be fleeting, but the ones who were vulnerable will stay with me. Always it will be the spirit that was important. Those who showed themselves to me.

I will cling to beauty. The images will be of the sea. Music will have healed pain.

All the dresses will have been unimportant.

Even the striving will be unimportant. What will resonate will only be where I surrendered to love, to the moment.

It will have been important to be kind to everyone.

Those who were consistent. And the times that I surprised myself by being so myself.

Sexual feelings, all of them, not necessarily in bed, but sexual feeling for people I was talking to, I will remember all that brightly.

The pristineness of the sun on the sea.

Hot summer nights, walking.

Phone messages that excited me. I won't remember the words or the issues, but I will remember the pleasure of connection.

Anyone who graced the passage of time with humor.

So many people, it will seem, needed love. It will seem like it had been impossible to give all that was needed.

The consistency of friendship. The long ones that endured everything. What we went through will be irrelevant and not even memorable, just that we did it together.

My lover taking the time to wake me up in the morning.

The closeness of talking and running an arm around a friend's neck, in friendship, in the sun.

Making calls and efforts for friends. Any effort. Any chance at love.

And what was all that busyness of making money? Perhaps only more of an opportunity to be in love relationships.

For some, the output of their work helps humanity. It was never such for me. I supported those who were feeding the cog. And that in itself was a privilege.

Friends' faces as they loved and were loved. It was such a mistake to put anxieties first.

The sensual joy of concentrating.